The
QA GUIDE

A Resource for Hospital
Quality Assurance

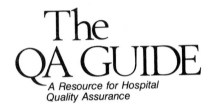

The
QA GUIDE
*A Resource for Hospital
Quality Assurance*

Authors: Karen Orloff Kaplan, MSW, MPH
Julie M. Hopkins, MA

Editor: Maryanne Shanahan

Contributors: Regina Walczak, MPH; James S. Roberts, MD; Francis C.
Dimond, Jr, MD; Jeffery Perlman, MD; Dale N. Schumacher, MD,
MEd; John Williamson, MD

Reviewers: William Andrews, MHA; Margaret D'Ambrosia, MBA; E. Martin
Egelston, PhD; James E. Grogan, PhD; Mary F. Kordick, RN;
Suzanne Miller, MPH; John E. Milton, FACHA; William Mudd,
MPH; LJ Nagel, MS; James P. Reber, MHA; Claire Tabel

Editorial and Design Staff: Maureen O'Brien; JoAnn Ballwanz; Denise M.
Heimlich; Robert R. Redman, MA; Donavan E. Vicha

Cover Design: Moira & Company

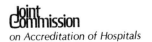
on Accreditation of Hospitals

63412

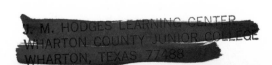

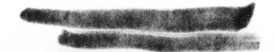

Foreword

Throughout its history, the Joint Commission on Accreditation of Hospitals (JCAH) has been dedicated to the goal of promoting optimal health care. This commitment is demonstrated in the approval of the new quality assurance standard for hospitals, which reflects the dynamic growth and change that is occurring in the field of quality assurance. The standard affords hospitals considerable flexibility in the manner in which they implement and administer their quality assurance programs and encourages innovation. The JCAH believes that such flexibility and innovation will encourage advancement in the state of the art of quality assurance.

The QA Guide: A Resource for Hospital Quality Assurance, 1980 edition, is intended as a guide to the current state of the art of quality assurance. Although it references JCAH's quality assurance standard for hospitals, the *Guide* should not be construed as JCAH's definitive statement on compliance with the standard. Rather, the *Guide* has been designed to help hospital staff organize a hospital-wide quality assurance program, focus evaluation activities on the identification and resolution of important problems in the provision of care, and incorporate quality assurance activities within the management decision-making process.

Because the state of the art of quality assurance will continue to evolve, JCAH will continue to test, revise, update, and improve our educational materials on quality assurance. The JCAH looks forward to advances in the field of quality assurance that will assist staff in making such improvements. We encourage your participation by asking you to inform us of your experiences, your approaches to quality assurance, and your suggestions.

John E. Affeldt, MD
President

Contents

Introduction

The increase in medical knowledge, the increasing sophistication of medical technology, the growing complexity of hospital services, and the rapid emergence of new health care professions have changed the complexion of health care delivery in the United States. Diagnostic and treatment procedures have become more complex; and the level of education of the American public has improved dramatically, contributing to greater awareness of and expectations from the health care field. Third-party payers have assumed an active, vocal role in health care financing and reimbursement; and federal financing of the care provided to large segments of the population has made hospitals and private physicians increasingly responsible and accountable to government and to society. An unprecedented inflation in the cost of care and in the utilization of services has occurred; public financing has been initiated; and federal attention to utilization review, cost containment, and mechanisms to evaluate quality has increased. In 1972, Congress directed the Department of Health, Education, and Welfare to develop its own program to ensure the necessity, quality, and cost-effectiveness of care financed under federal health care programs. Through this legislation, Professional Standards Review Organizations (PSROs) were established.

The JCAH and Quality Assurance

Throughout this period, health care professionals have maintained their dedication to improving the quality of patient care. This commitment is reflected in the standards and accreditation processes of the Joint Commission on Accreditation of Hospitals (JCAH).

Since its establishment in 1951 and during this period of rapid growth and change in the health care field, JCAH has emphasized quality and stressed the value of ongoing review and evaluation of care by medical and other professional staffs. Over the years, various means of reviewing and evaluating care have been recognized by JCAH. In 1972, JCAH developed an audit methodology designed to assist hospitals to objectively review and evaluate patient care, established a requirement for medical audits, and, in 1974, specified the number of audits to be performed.

Requirements Reconsidered

Although the establishment of numerical requirements was initially seen as an overwhelming task involving extensive paperwork, health care professionals responded to the requirements. They recognized the value of reviewing quality of patient care, if not the value of conducting extensive audits. In the period of questioning that typically accompanies any new procedure or requirement, both JCAH and the health care professionals who were evaluating care began to realize that medical audit requirements were self-limiting: Adherence to numerical requirements limited the amount and scope of care evaluated. In addition, emphasis on broad diagnosis-based review specified by the JCAH methodology encouraged hospitals to focus only on diagnostic topics rather than on identified or potential problems in patient care or clinical performance. Other quality assessment and quality related activities (eg, review of nursing care and support services; tissue, antibiotic, and blood utilization review; delineation of clinical privileges; and monitoring of clinical practice) were not coordinated with audit activities or recognized as part of an overall quality assurance program.

As hospitals attempted to evaluate care and meet requirements—and, indeed, some hospitals demonstrated impressive results in the evaluation and improvement of care—survey findings demonstrated that patient care and clinical performance had not improved to the extent anticipated. In some cases, changes in patient care and clinical performance were not in proportion to the amount of time invested and the costs associated with audit activity. Evaluation of the quality of patient care had evolved to the point at which a wider perspective, which took into account all hospital activities contributing to patient care, had to be pursued.

These factors were important considerations in the JCAH decision to eliminate the numerical audit requirement, effective April 1979, and to substantially revise the approach to quality assurance requirements. The "new" quality assurance standard for hospitals is designed to help health care professionals develop a more sophisticated, comprehensive approach to quality assurance activities. The factors which precipitated a healthy examination of the state of the art of quality assurance have influenced a more dynamic and useful quality assurance standard. The standard, which is effective for accreditation decision purposes on January 1, 1981,

- emphasizes the value of a coordinated, hospital-wide quality assurance program;

- allows greater flexibility in approaches to problem identification, assessment, and resolution;
- emphasizes the importance of focusing quality assurance activity on problems whose resolution will have a significant impact on patient care and outcomes;
- emphasizes the importance of focusing quality assurance activity on areas where demonstrable problem resolution is possible;
- encourages the use of multiple data sources to identify problems; and
- discourages the use of quality assurance studies only for the purpose of documenting high quality care.

The QA Guide: A Resource for Hospital Quality Assurance

The QA Guide is designed to help hospitals meet the intent of the quality assurance standard and to develop and implement comprehensive, problem-focused approaches to quality assurance that have a positive impact on the quality of patient care and clinical performance.

Comprehensive Quality Assurance Programs

The QA Guide addresses the importance of organizing a flexible quality assurance program that meets the unique needs of your hospital. To be maximally flexible, effective, and efficient, the quality assurance program should be planned carefully and quality assurance activities should be integrated to the degree possible. Planning a coordinated program involves detailed assessment of all quality assurance activities currently conducted in your hospital. Such an assessment should help identify the strengths and correct the weaknesses of present activities; and the program should stress integration and coordination of activities to encourage strong, useful interrelationships, enhance communication, and minimize duplication. A well-constructed quality assurance program allows approaches to problem solving that preserve the integrity of individual disciplines and their unique quality assurance efforts while providing for appropriate sharing of information.

The first five chapters of the *Guide* should help you to assess your current activities and organize an effective, comprehensive quality assurance program. The *Guide* will assist you to

- set goals and objectives for quality assurance;
- assess current quality assurance activities;
- analyze assessment results;
- use assessment results as a basis for organizing the hospital-wide quality assurance program;

- develop a quality assurance plan; and
- implement the quality assurance program.

Problem-Focused Approach

The new quality assurance standard requires a problem-focused approach to quality assurance activity. The interpretation of the standard states that "to obtain maximal benefit, any approach to quality assurance must focus on the resolution of known or suspected problems (that impact directly or indirectly on patients) or, when indicated, on areas with potential for substantial improvements in patient care."* A quality assurance program that results in problem resolution depends on explicit, knowledgeable use of a logical approach to problem solving. The following basic components of quality assurance activity constitute a logical approach to problem solving:

- identify problems;
- determine priorities for problem assessment and problem resolution;
- establish clinically valid criteria and select appropriate assessment methods;
- establish problem causes most amenable to correction and plan and implement corrective actions; and
- evaluate and monitor problem resolution.

Any quality assurance activity, whether simple or complex, should be based on the problem-solving logic delineated above. However, these five components are *not* steps that must be rigidly followed to meet accreditation requirements or rules that outline the "right" or the "only" approach to quality assurance, nor do these components imply that new forms for quality assurance activities are in the offing. The five components of quality assurance activity *are* a set of guidelines for quality assessment that are based on logical principles of evaluation and that are most likely implicit (ie, not written) in many quality assurance activities already. However, the components should become an explicit part of the hospital's quality assurance activities because, when clearly spelled out and acknowledged, they can be used to evaluate whether the program is planned and implemented effectively. Flexibility in the depth and speed of application of the components is both appropriate and acceptable; that is, although the components should be considered in problem solving, it is not necessary to isolate and apply each component in a strict methodological sense.

Chapters 6-10 of the *Guide* discuss the components of a problem-focused approach to quality assurance and will assist you to

- use multiple data sources for problem identification;

Accreditation Manual for Hospitals, 1981 Edition. Chicago: JCAH, 1980, p 151.

- determine priorities for problem assessment and resolution;
- select and implement appropriate assessment methods;
- establish clinically valid criteria; and
- select appropriate sample sizes.

A comprehensive problem-focused approach to quality assurance will only be successful if identified problems are resolved and if resolution of problems is sustained. The impact of the program on patient care and clinical performance should be assessed, and the effectiveness of the overall program should be evaluated on a regular basis. Chapter 11 discusses annual reevaluation of the program and suggests questions that might be useful in assessing the results of your hospital's quality assurance activities.

Comment

Review and evaluation of patient care is a dynamic process that offers exciting opportunities for achieving and maintaining optimal quality of care in hospitals. Staff of JCAH invite you to participate in this process by using *The QA Guide: A Resource for Hospital Quality Assurance* in the spirit in which it is written—as a resource and guide for developing and implementing effective mechanisms for evaluating and improving the quality of patient care in your hospital.

Chapter 1. Planning a Quality Assurance Program

Quality isn't method. It's the goal toward which method is aimed. *

Pirsig

The following distinction between methods and goals will help you establish an effective quality assurance program in your hospital: Methods change constantly; goals usually remain the same. You change methods to improve your chances of attaining goals. The process is ongoing and dynamic, involving constant change, correction, and improvement. As progress is made and objectives met, the focus of the process shifts to greater improvement or to other areas in need of attention. The management of this dynamic process is the purpose of your quality assurance program. Providing the optimal quality of care within available resources is the inherent goal of your quality assurance program. Numerous methods are discussed in this *Guide*. Use those that seem appropriate to your hospital, but don't hesitate to change methods that don't work.

The commitment of hospital leadership is essential to the success of any hospital's quality assurance program. Without commitment from the top, other staff will most likely consider the program a nuisance, a paper exercise performed to satisfy external agencies. On the other hand, if hospital leaders are committed to and express support for the program, if they treat quality assurance as a priority, and if they use quality assurance information as a basis for their activities and decisions, then the program will most likely succeed. Other hospital staff will support it, and the quality assurance program could become the basis for management decisions throughout the hospital.

Responsibility for planning can be assigned to an individual (eg, an assistant administrator, a director of medical education), or a group (eg, a task force comprised of several top managers). Whoever is given re-

---

*Pirsig, RM: *Zen and the Art of Motorcycle Maintenance: An Inquiry Into Values.* Toronto: Bantam Books, 1974.

sponsibility for planning should obtain extensive input from staff, particularly from individuals actively involved in quality assurance activities. Key members of the medical staff should be consulted throughout the planning process. By including staff in the planning process, you increase their acceptance and support of the program, and you will probably find it easier to obtain their help should you need it in the future. Extensive staff participation also provides for a variety of perspectives in the planning process.

The importance of planning to an effective quality assurance program cannot be overemphasized. Careful planning is the cornerstone of any good program: It secures and strengthens the various components of the program, and, at the same time, it guides and supports staff in their attempts to achieve the objectives and goals of the program. Planning begins when the purpose of the program, and the means or methods of achieving the purpose are written as program goals and objectives.

Goals are general results or conditions that you expect to achieve. Specify goals in measurable terms and in a statement of relatively broad scope. Goals should guide you in developing objectives. Objectives are similar to goals in that they are also stated in terms that will serve as measurable indices of progress. They are different from goals in that they are narrower and more specific in scope, and they are related to the eventual achievement of a goal. The difference between goals and objectives is illustrated by the following example. A hospital's goal is to provide high quality care; one of its objectives is to comply with JCAH standards. Successful compliance with these standards, will contribute to attainment of the goal—high quality care.

The mission statement of your hospital is a useful resource in determining goals. Statements concerning the proper utilization of resources, reduced liability, and a safe patient environment relate to achievable, optimal conditions that can serve as goals for a quality assurance program. Once you have stated the goals, you may want to incorporate them into a statement of purpose. This statement can be incorporated into the written plan describing your quality assurance program.

Objectives should also be written. Unlike goals, which usually remain the same, objectives may change periodically and new objectives set as others are achieved. Written objectives should be specific and should include the date by which the objective is expected to be met. For instance, if one of your objectives is "to develop a promotional campaign that explains the quality assurance program to all staff," add the date you expect to launch the campaign (eg, March 1980).

Objectives can apply to the entire institution or to one of its departments. For example, a hospital-wide objective might be "to orient all department directors to their roles in the quality assurance program by April 1980." A departmental objective for nursing services might be "to assess the administration of medications quarterly and reduce errors by 10%."

Chapter 2. Assessing Quality Assurance Activities

Determining the status of current quality assurance activities is the second step in planning a hospital-wide quality assurance program. This assessment is conducted to identify the scope, purpose, and effectiveness of current activities; to ascertain whether such activities meet all JCAH requirements for review and evaluation; to identify strengths and weaknesses in the overall quality assurance program; to determine whether duplication in activity, overlap in authority and responsibility, or unnecessary expenditures in staff time and resources exist; and to determine whether expansion, reorganization, or streamlining of the current program is necessary and appropriate.

Included in the assessment should be medical staff functions such as departmental meetings, continuing medical education, and credentialing; departmental activities such as emergency services, nursing, and anesthesiology reviews; and hospital-wide activities such as risk control, safety programs, and infection control. Although difficult, it might be useful to identify the cost and time spent in the conduct of quality assurance activities. The cost of an activity might be measured by calculating the number of man-hours spent in meetings and in data preparation and then multiplying those hours by a predetermined dollar value. Costs can also be determined by calculating the number of man-hours and multiplying that number by the hourly salary of paid personnel. However, the latter approach does not account for the time and cost of non-salaried committee members.

You might wish to estimate the productivity or effectiveness of a quality assurance activity by viewing the impact of the activity on care in relation to the time, effort, and dollars expended. This approach tends to be subjective but can prove helpful by identifying areas in which changes may be indicated.

Assessment Tools

To assist you in assessing your current quality assurance activities, ten questions and instructions for answering each question are provided on pages 4-8. These questions are not necessarily all-inclusive, and their use need not be limited only to an initial assessment of the quality assurance program. That is, you might wish to use or incorporate questions from other sources (such as the *Hospital Survey Profile,* the *Program on Hospital Accreditation Standards (PHAS) Manual,* and/or the evaluation questions in Chapter 11, pages 129-131) in your periodic and/or annual evaluations of the quality assurance program. A table of organization of quality assurance activities is also a useful tool in your hospital. This chart should identify all functions, committees, and departmental activities related to quality assurance, illustrate the relationship among activities, and depict the reporting relationships.

Although only one person might be assigned to conduct the assessment, others necessarily will be consulted. Each department or committee might be requested to complete the questions for the activity for which it is responsible. In such instances, assign someone knowledgeable about overall quality assurance requirements (eg, an assistant administrator or committee chairman) to work with the departments or committees during assessment.

When each assessment question has been answered for each quality assurance activity, you might wish to display the results on a matrix to facilitate analysis of the information. (For an example of an assessment matrix which you might wish to use or modify, see pages 6-7.)

Initial Assessment Questions

Respond to each of the following ten questions for each quality assurance activity conducted in your institution. In instances where the question does not apply to a particular function, indicate that it is not applicable.

1. Is the function performed by an individual or committee? Name the individual/committee that performs that function. For example, utilization review (UR) may be handled by both a UR coordinator and a UR committee. Both should be indicated.

2. Who is routinely responsible for the function? Indicate the responsible person or position, and/or the individual who coordinates the function on a full-time or part-time basis.

3. Is there a written description or procedure for the function? Indicate if a written description or procedure for the function exists. An attached copy of the description or procedure can be useful in analyzing the function.

4. What data sources are used to perform this function? List the data sources used for each function. Data sources may include, but need not be limited to, one or a combination of the following:

- medical records;
- morbidity/mortality review;
- review of prescriptions;
- profile analysis, including PSRO and other regional data;
- specific process-oriented/outcome-oriented studies;
- incident reports;
- laboratory, radiologic, and other diagnostic clinical reports;
- financial data (eg, hospital charge data for services rendered, malpractice claims experience);
- utilization review findings;
- data from staff interviews and observation of hospital activities;
- patient surveys or comments; and
- data originating from third-party payers/fiscal intermediaries.

5. Are preestablished, clinically valid criteria used? Clinically valid criteria are statements about the structure, process, or outcome of care drawn from the best in knowledge and experience of experts and from the health care literature. Some quality assurance functions, such as continuing education, may use objectives or standards of care and of clinical performance as appropriate measures.

6. If a purpose of the function is to identify problems, are important problems identified? If problem identification is a purpose of the function, indicate if a projection is made of the problem's impact on patients (ie, those problems which, if allowed to continue unresolved, are likely to have an impact on patient care and clinical performance). For example, are incident reports on medication errors analyzed to determine the scope and cause of a pattern or increased number of events, or are they merely tabulated?

7. Does the responsible individual or committee recommend or implement action? If the responsible individual/committee refers action to another committee, it recommends action; if the individual/committee is responsible for taking action, it implements action. Some committees such as the medical staff executive committee can recommend *and* implement action.

8. Is there monitoring to determine effectiveness of action? Monitoring means that assessment is done to determine if the problem(s) was corrected or improved as a result of the action taken. Monitoring (follow-up) may be accomplished by:

- performing a new study using the same, new, and/or revised criteria;
- reviewing data collected after corrective action is instituted;
- directly observing the activity or personnel being assessed; and
- interviewing pertinent personnel and/or patients.

Assessment Questions	Credentialing	Clinical Department Review	Tissue/Surgical Case Review and Evaluation	Morbidity/Mortality	Pharmacy and Therapeutics	Blood Utilization Review and Evaluation	Antibiotic U and
1. Is the function performed by an individual or committee?							
2. Who is routinely responsible for the function?							
3. Is there a written description or procedure for the function?							
4. What data sources are used to perform this function?							
5. Are preestablished, clinically valid criteria used?							
6. If a purpose of the function is to identify problems, are important problems identified?							
7. Does the responsible individual or committee recommend or implement action?							
8. Is there monitoring to determine effectiveness of action?							
9. To whom are the results of the function reported? With whom are they shared?							
10. Is the function evaluated routinely?							

Review / ...aluation	Review and Evaluation of Support Services	Audit	Infection Control	Safety	Utilization Review	Risk Control	Continuing Education	Accreditation	Patient Representative Information	

9. To whom are the results of the function reported? With whom are they shared? Indicate the committee or individual to whom the results of the function must be routinely directed. For example, utilization review findings might be directed to the medical executive committee, the chief of staff, the chief executive officer, and the governing body.

Also indicate any other functions with which results are shared. Sharing the results/findings of quality assurance functions might be accomplished by circulating minutes, memos, and/or newsletters to any other function. For example, infection control findings might be shared with the pharmacy and therapeutics committee, the director of nursing, and the director of the department of surgery.

10. Is the function evaluated routinely? Reappraisal of the overall quality assurance program at least annually is a requirement of the quality assurance standard. Review of the individual functions of a quality assurance program is recommended as an effective means of reappraising the entire quality assurance effort (see Chapter 11).

Chapter 3. Analyzing Assessment Results

Analyzing initial assessment results constitutes the third step in planning your quality assurance program. This analysis should help you to identify activities that are performed effectively; to identify activities that need improvement or restructuring; to determine whether duplication exists among activities; to determine whether lines of authority, accountability, and reporting are clear; to determine what steps should be taken toward integration and coordination of activities; and to determine necessary alterations in the organization of and procedures for quality assurance activities.

If you used the ten questions in Chapter 2 to assess your current quality assurance activities, the information and questions in this chapter will help you to analyze the data gathered during the initial assessment described in Chapter 2. Each of the ten questions from Chapter 2 is presented, and the additional questions which follow are designed to assist you to look at each quality assurance activity individually (see pages 10-13) and at patterns which cross all activities (see pages 13-18). Looking at patterns across all activities should help you refine your current program to meet requirements for coordination and communication. Because this analysis across activities should identify necessary changes in the structure and organization of the quality assurance program, it should be conducted by key decision-makers in the facility or by the task force/ committee which was responsible for setting goals and objectives for the program.

If you have constructed a table of organization that depicts current quality assurance activities, analysis of that table should help you identify whether the approach to current quality assurance activities is systematic; whether lines of authority and accountability for quality assurance are clearly defined; whether coordination and integration of activities occurs in some areas; whether any one committee or individual handles the major portion of quality assurance activities; and whether duplication of effort exists.

Assessment Analysis Questions: Individual Activities

1. Is the function performed by an individual or committee? Assessment of your response to this question is intended to show whether an individual, a committee, or both are necessary and/or sufficient to perform quality assurance-related duties throughout the hospital, and what modifications might be initiated to strive for more efficient use of staff time and resources.

If an individual or committee performs each function,

- are all the duties associated with the function completed in the specified time frames?
- are other assignments not related to this function neglected in order to fulfill this obligation?
- does the function review care that is representative of the discipline it encompasses?

If an individual and a committee perform a function,

- does each have distinct responsibilities?
- are both necessary to complete the function in terms of time and cost?

2. Who is routinely responsible for the function? Assessment of your response to this question is intended to indicate whether assignment of responsibility is appropriate and whether authority and accountability have been defined.

- Does the individual have the appropriate knowledge and skills to perform the duties of the function?
- Is the individual responsible for the function the same person to whom any hospital-wide questions about the function are directed?
- Does this individual have responsibility for ascertaining that all procedures in the function are performed in a timely manner?

3. Is there a written description or procedure for the function? Assessment of your response to this question is intended to determine if guidelines for the function exist and if they are adequate or need improvement.

- If the individual responsible for performing this function were to leave, would another individual be able to perform the function based on the description?
- Does the description include purpose and/or objectives, responsibilities, use of criteria, mechanisms for feedback of results to practitioners, reporting relationships, means of interacting with other quality assurance functions, and procedures for evaluation of the function?

4. What data sources are used to perform this function? Assessment of your response to this question is intended to determine whether the data sources used are sufficient.

- Is only a single data source used for the function?
- What other data sources might be used to identify or solve problems associated with this function? For example, to complete the antibiotic review function, would it be helpful to examine pharmacy reports, laboratory reports, and medication error reports?

5. Are preestablished, clinically valid criteria used? Assessment of your response to this question is intended to indicate whether preestablished criteria, objectives, or standards are used, when appropriate, to measure attainment of goals.

- Are objectives, standards, or criteria based on a review of clinical literature?
- Are they agreed upon by the staff and/or does the chairman of the committee accept responsibility for their reasonableness?
- Are criteria frequently changed because of the staff's difference of opinion about their validity? Are they changed to conform with current hospital practice, thereby undermining their usefulness in identifying problems in patient care or clinical performance?
- Are there any difficulties in establishing criteria?

6. If a purpose of the function is to identify problems, are important problems identified? Assessment of your response to this question is intended to indicate whether the function is responsible for identifying problems and whether it identifies problems that have an impact on patient care and clinical performance.

- Are problems in patient care rarely identified? Is lack of documentation the primary or sole problem identified?
- Are priorities set for assessment or resolution of identified problems?
- Will resolution of problems that have been identified have an impact on patient care? (Examples of results of improved patient care might be decreased mortality or infection rates; decreased incidence of transfusion reactions, patient falls, or unnecessary surgery; and decreased length of stay.)

7. Does the responsible individual or committee recommend or implement action? Assessment of your response to this question is intended to determine if action is taken to resolve problems in an efficient manner.

If the individual or committee recommends actions,

- are the recommendations clear and specific, and do they lead to correction of the problem?
- are the recommendations forwarded to an individual or group that has authority to take action?
- are recommended actions implemented by the individual or group to whom they are referred?

- is feedback on corrective actions provided to the committee that initiated recommendations?

If the individual or committee only implements actions,

- are recommendations routinely received by the individual or committee?
- are recommendations clear and specific?
- are actions implemented on a timely basis? If not, why?
- do the actions taken lead to correction of the problem?

If the individual or committee recommends and implements action,

- are actions implemented on a timely basis?
- does the individual or committee appear to be overburdened?
- do the actions taken lead to correction of the problem?

8. Is there monitoring to determine effectiveness of action? Assessment of your response to this question is intended to determine whether effectiveness of action is assessed and whether sustained resolution of the problem is achieved.

- Are implemented actions effective? For example, do they result in desired changes in compliance, incident rates, policies, or procedures?
- If not, does the individual or committee understand the importance of monitoring (follow-up), have a mechanism to conduct monitoring, and assign responsibilities and time frames for monitoring?
- After implemented actions are shown to be effective, does the individual or committee periodically reassess the problem to see that resolution is sustained?

9. To whom are the results of the function reported? With whom are they shared? Assessment of your response to this question is intended to determine the adequacy of information reporting and sharing.

- Are findings of the function reported, as appropriate, to the medical staff, chief executive officer, and governing body through a designated mechanism?
- Are findings that relate to care provided by a clinical unit which is not represented by the function made available to the director of that unit? For example, if blood utilization studies show inappropriate blood ordering and/or usage for surgery, is the chief of surgery notified?
- What other quality assurance functions receive results/findings of this function?

10. Is the function evaluated routinely? Assessment of your response to this question is intended to determine whether the function is effective as demonstrated by evaluation of the function in relation to the overall quality assurance program.

- Are the roles and effectiveness of the function evaluated at least annually?
- Are procedures instituted, altered, or deleted as a result of evaluation?

- Is the function evaluated for impact on patient care and/or clinical performance?
- Are time, cost, and resources considered in the evaluation?

Assessment Analysis Questions: Across Activities

1. Is the function performed by an individual or committee? A major intent of the quality assurance standard is that hospitals institute a plan for assuring the comprehensiveness and integration of an overall quality assurance program. To accomplish this, individuals or committees must be designated to perform certain functions, and efforts must be made to eliminate unnecessary duplication.

If analysis across functions shows that tasks are either not completed or are not completed on time, consider whether adequate personnel or resources have been allocated to accomplish each function. Likewise, if tasks are completed at the expense of other duties performed by these individuals or committees, reconsider how personnel are used.

2. Who is routinely responsible for the function? According to the interpretation of the quality assurance standard, responsibility for various quality assurance functions must be defined in writing. If analysis across functions indicates a problem about who is responsible for quality assurance functions, consider whether designation of such responsibility is lacking in the written description of each function or whether the scope of responsibility needs to be explained more clearly. Also consider whether the individuals assigned responsibilities possess appropriate knowledge and skills to fulfill their tasks. For example, assigning primary responsibility for a medical staff function (ie, setting clinical criteria for an audit) to the medical record department is inappropriate.

As you attempt to integrate your quality assurance program, you might consider whether one individual or committee could assume primary responsibility for overseeing all other quality assurance functions. A central committee or individual could undertake responsibilities to ascertain that other committees identify and assess problems, act to resolve problems, and report findings/results to appropriate groups. A central mechanism could also keep track of whether tasks are completed in a timely manner. Types of organization, including coordination by a staff person, committee, or department are discussed in Chapter 4.

3. Is there a written description or procedures for the function? The quality assurance standard interpretation states: "The plan for assuring the comprehensiveness and integration of the overall quality assurance program and for delegating responsibility for the various activities that contribute to quality assurance must be defined in writing."*

Accreditation Manual for Hospitals, 1981 Edition. Chicago: JCAH, 1980, p 151.

If written procedures do not exist (particularly for those functions clearly specified in medical staff bylaws, rules and regulations), they should be developed to delineate the purpose of each function and define its place within a comprehensive quality assurance program. Consider including the following items in your written procedures: purpose, responsibilities, reporting relationships, specifications for interacting with other quality assurance functions, and procedures for evaluating the function.

If written procedures do exist, are they complete and current? For example, if you plan to appoint an individual and assign authority for implementing action, this change should be reflected in your written procedures. Consider modifying procedures to reflect changes in the function that you may wish to make, as well as changes necessary to integrate functions within a comprehensive quality assurance program.

4. What data sources are used to perform this function? Although the medical record remains an important data source in problem identification, the interpretation of the quality assurance standard suggests other potentially useful sources. If a single data source is used, consider the potential benefits in expanding the data base used to complete that function. For example, in mortality review you may also wish to examine comparative data of mortality rates on both a regional and national basis. Consider the organizational channels that are necessary to ascertain that this information is received routinely.

If multiple data sources are used, consider whether difficulties exist in obtaining information. For example, if infection control review requires use of microbiology, laboratory, and/or pharmacy reports, is this information routinely available? If not, should access to this information be improved?

Regardless of whether single or multiple sources are used, consider whether data retrieval activities are duplicated. For example, are the same medical records being used in separate medical staff, nursing, and physical therapy studies of hip fracture? Consider whether a central coordination mechanism (ie, individual, department, or committee) might discover this duplication and recommend an intradisciplinary study.

5. Are preestablished, clinically valid criteria used? The interpretation of the quality assurance standard states: "Written criteria that relate to essential or critical aspects of patient care and that are generally acceptable to the clinical staffs shall be used to assess problems and measure compliance with achievable goals."* Failure to use preestablished and generally accepted measures may result in such problems as different measures being used by different departments, conformity to an unacceptable or undesired standard, subjective assessment, or establishment of unachievable goals.

Clinically valid criteria, objectives, and/or standards should be based on a review of the literature and other resources. Consider whether use

---

Accreditation Manual for Hospitals, 1981 Edition. Chicago: JCAH, 1980, p 152.

of a single, clinically valid criterion, in some instances, may avoid unnecessary duplication of work and provide information for several functions. For example, a single criterion such as "operation for perforation, laceration, tear, or injury of an organ incurred during an invasive procedure" could provide information useful to hospital legal counsel and to the functions of risk control, surgical case review, patient representation, utilization review, continuing education, and credentialing.

6. If a purpose of the function is to identify problems, are important problems identified? Another major intent of the quality assurance standard is to focus review of patient care on identified problems and to set appropriate priorities for their assessment and resolution. If identification of important problems is difficult across functions, consider whether it is necessary to redirect the objectives of the function. For example, studies might examine specific problems (such as wound infections in general surgery) as opposed to diagnostic topics (such as cholecystectomy). Determine whether access to additional data sources might make the function more productive.

Also, consider if an individual, department, or committee could facilitate setting priorities for problem assessment and resolution through central screening and dissemination of data. For example, a central committee might note that antibiotic review, pharmacy and therapeutics review, and incident reports of adverse drug reactions show misuse of a toxic and expensive medication. Each of these review functions might be unaware of the findings of the other committees. Based on the extent of the problem, a centralized committee, or a department or individual, might determine that assessment and resolution of this problem is a high priority.

7. Does the responsible individual or committee recommend or implement action? An essential component of a sound quality assurance program is the implementation of action appropriate to resolution of the problem. If recommendations and implementation of actions are not accomplished across functions, consider whether responsibility for this task is unclear or has not been delegated appropriately. For example, responsibility may be lacking for action recommendation and implementation or those with authority may not be fulfilling their obligations; if so, this problem should be corrected.

If action implementation is a problem across functions, perhaps this indicates that the individuals or committees are unsure of how to determine effective actions pertinent to the problems or that authority for taking action has not been delegated. For instance, notifying practitioners about the existence of a problem by sending a letter or offering a continuing education program may not be the best approach for all problems. Other types of action that are specific to the cause of the problem could be explored. To give a more specific example, let us say that surgical case review indicated a high incidence of fixation loss following hip surgery performed by one physician. Appropriate actions might be to require the physician to consult with other surgeons on operative technique and/or to have the chief of orthopedics attend subsequent operations performed by the practitioner.

Another reason for lack of recommendation or implementation of actions could be that the responsible individual or committee is overburdened. If so, consider whether a redistribution and/or centralization of responsibilities with another individual, group, or committee would be appropriate. Consider also whether delegation of authority has been lacking and needs to be delineated. This problem frequently can be eliminated by assigning an individual to monitor the status of recommended action to assure implementation of that action within the specified time frame.

8. Is there monitoring to determine effectiveness of action? Use of monitoring to assure that the desired result of an action has been achieved and sustained is an essential component of a sound quality assurance program. Failure to assess actions prevents you from determining their appropriateness and from determining whether actual improvements in patient care and clinical performance have occurred. In addition, unless you know that actions are effective and appropriate, resources spent to correct the problem may have been wasted.

If analysis revealed that monitoring was not performed across functions, perhaps responsibility for this task has not been delegated or written procedures do not exist. If so, develop procedures for monitoring that specify how follow-up should be accomplished and assign the individual or committee responsible for monitoring.

If you discover that actual improvements in patient care or clinical performance do not occur as a result of recommended action (eg, no change in incident rates or in compliance with procedures and policies), you should evaluate whether the action was appropriate to the problem. For example, the action chosen to correct the problem of a high rate of urinary tract infection (UTI) may have been a continuing education program for nurses on management of UTI. If subsequent monitoring failed to show a decrease in the rate of UTI, perhaps the action was inappropriate to the problem. Instruction on prevention of UTIs and Foley catheter care may have been more appropriate.

Actions taken to resolve problems may result in only a temporary improvement. For example, to resolve the problem of a high rate of patient falls, policies were written requiring the use of side rails on beds. Several months after implementation of this action and compliance by the nursing staff, incident reports revealed that patient falls were again occurring at a high rate. Analysis to determine the cause of the problem revealed that new personnel had not been made aware of the policy. Action was then taken to assure appropriate orientation of new staff to existing policies and procedures.

9. To whom are the results of the function reported? With whom are they shared? As the interpretation of the quality assurance standard states, "Pertinent findings of quality assurance activities throughout the hospital shall be reported to one, two, or all of the following as appropriate, through their designated mechanisms: the medical staff, the chief executive officer, and the governing body."* Furthermore, the interpretation suggests that communication may be enhanced and potential cost savings may be realized through coordination of quality assurance functions and information sharing.

If analysis revealed that information reporting was not performed across functions, perhaps responsibility for this task has not been delegated or written procedures do not exist. If so, develop procedures for information sharing and specify the individual or committee responsible for this task. If not, perhaps duplication of effort is occurring. For example, blood utilization review, surgical review, medical audit of a surgical topic, and morbidity/mortality review all reveal a problem with transfusion reactions. If each of these functions investigates the same problem in isolation, costly duplication of effort is likely to occur. Information-sharing may pinpoint such duplication and lead to more efficient use of resources through a single investigation and resolution of the problem.

If information on problems, findings, and actions is being channeled primarily to one individual or committee, you might wish to consider whether this individual or committee could serve as a clearinghouse for all quality assurance functions. This would integrate the task of information-sharing and might assure that all problems, findings, and actions are routinely disseminated to appropriate individuals or committees. If a mechanism exists to facilitate sharing of data sources, this same body may be the one to coordinate information-sharing.

10. Is the function evaluated routinely? The interpretation of the quality assurance standard requires reappraisal of the hospital's quality assurance program at least annually. This task can perhaps best be accomplished if the effectiveness of each function within the overall program is ascertained.

If analysis across functions reveals that evaluation is not being done, perhaps responsibility for this task has not been delegated or written procedures do not exist. If so, develop procedures for evaluation and specify the individual or committee responsible for this task.

Evaluation of a comprehensive quality assurance program could be enhanced by examination of the purpose of each function within the program, by the function's ability to identify problems that will have an impact on patient care and clinical performance through the establishment of priorities for problem assessment and resolution, and by the effectiveness of actions taken to assure sustained resolution. Presumably, reappraisal will identify specific components of the quality assurance program that need to be instituted, altered, or deleted. For example, a hospital's time and cost studies revealed that costly data retrieval time was used to gather records for an extensive audit of appendectomy in which the most significant finding was a high incidence of wound infection.

Accreditation Manual for Hospitals, 1981 Edition. Chicago: JCAH, 1980, p 153.

The surgical review committee at the hospital routinely compiles data on incidence of wound infection for the most commonly performed surgical procedures. Analyzing this situation, the committee responsible for evaluation of the quality assurance program suggested that the surgical review committee share its reports on incidence with other committees, including the medical audit committee. Furthermore, the evaluation body recommended that, in the future, the medical audit committee utilize surgical review information as one way to identify surgical problems.

Chapter 4. Organizing a Quality Assurance Program

Before you begin to organize your hospital's quality assurance program, you should realize that JCAH does not require hospitals to establish new committees to comply with its quality assurance standard. Staff of many hospitals believe that they have to establish a committee to perform each function required by JCAH standards; however, the *Accreditation Manual for Hospitals* actually requires only four committees: an executive committee of the governing body, an executive committee of the medical staff, a hospital-wide infection control committee, and a hospital-wide safety committee.* And, in small nondepartmentalized hospitals with approximately 15 or less active medical staff members, the functions of the medical staff executive committee may be performed by the medical staff as a whole. Generally, the standards require certain functions to be performed, such as surgical case or antibiotic review, but these functions do not have to be carried out by committees. The knowledge that JCAH is more concerned with functions being performed than with committees being established may assist you in understanding the standards and in organizing your quality assurance program.

The quality assurance standard clearly identifies responsibility within hospital quality assurance programs: "It is the governing body's responsibility to establish, maintain, and support, through the hospital's administration and medical staff, an ongoing quality assurance program. . . ."† The standard also states that "Each clinical discipline is responsible for identifying and resolving problems related to patient

---

*The *Accreditation Manual for Hospitals* also addresses the following functions:
  Planning: Institutional planning can be performed by an existing committee that includes governing body, administration, and medical staff membership.
  Special care units: A multidisciplinary committee of the medical staff is required in multipurpose special care units only.
  Home care services: A multidisciplinary committee, including at least one physician and one registered nurse, is required. This can be an existing committee that includes the director of the home care program.
  †*Accreditation Manual for Hospitals, 1981 Edition.* Chicago: JCAH, 1980, p 151.

care. . . ."* (This aspect of the standard is further explained in the sections of the *AMH* that refer to particular disciplines, such as the sections regarding the medical staff, nursing services, and other professional services.) Thus, the governing body is ultimately responsible for establishing the quality assurance program; the administration and medical staff share the delegated responsibility for the program; and each clinical discipline is responsible for identifying and resolving problems related to the care they provide.

Review and evaluation requirements of the quality assurance standard are not new. What is new is that the reviews focus on problems and their resolution and that the results of review and evaluation activities must now be coordinated or integrated, to the degree possible, within a hospital-wide quality assurance program. This means that the results should be shared with the appropriate people to facilitate resolution of identified problems and that the review and evaluation is conducted efficiently and does not duplicate efforts. The quality assurance standard does not specify a preferred way of coordinating activities; every hospital has the flexibility necessary to design a system that is compatible with its existing activities.

Organizing for Coordination

Although several activities must be performed to coordinate quality assurance activities effectively, these activities do not have to be performed in any one place or by any one committee, group, or individual. However, authority and responsibility for each action should be clearly delineated. You must decide which individual, committee, or group can most effectively

- plan quality assurance activities;
- identify problems;
- collate, display, and disseminate data;
- set priorities for evaluation;
- analyze data;
- recommend action;
- take action; and
- monitor results.

Some or all of these activities could be accomplished by a committee, but in most hospitals they are accomplished by a committee or group working with an individual or department. This is because all activities involved in effective coordination are not performed at the same organizational level. For example, determining priorities for resolving prob-

---

Accreditation Manual for Hospitals, 1981 Edition. Chicago: JCAH, 1980, p 151.

lems and approving implementation of necessary actions might occur at the highest organizational level, while analyzing data and monitoring results may occur at the departmental or committee level. This does not mean that every action taken to resolve a problem must be approved by the medical staff executive committee, the chief executive officer, or the governing body, but they must be kept well-informed; and they should set priorities and approve actions for those problems that are critical to patient care and safety or that involve major expenditures or changes in staff.

Priorities can be set and actions approved through several different organizational arrangements. One hospital elected to designate the chief executive officer, chief of staff, director of nursing, and a member of the governing body to be the group responsible for decision-making. In another institution, recommended priorities and actions related to the medical staff are sent to the chief of the medical staff for approval, and recommendations related to the professional staff are sent to the chief executive officer for approval. (It should be noted that medical staff recommendations are approved by the medical staff executive committee in most hospitals.) A third hospital has department directors set priorities for resolution of problems in each of their areas. In yet another hospital, the joint conference committee is responsible for approving priorities and actions for all clinical staffs. Results of quality assurance activities are summarized by the administration and the medical staff executive committee and are sent to the joint conference committee. In any event, it is important to clearly specify who has authority for taking action and who has responsibility for intervening when a recommended action is not taken or when follow-up indicates that the action was not effective. Check your hospital and medical staff bylaws to determine if this responsibility has already been designated to a committee, group, or individual. In your analysis of current activities, you may already have identified who is currently making the decisions and can determine if that decision-making authority is at the appropriate level.

Other coordination activities can be divided among committees, departments, or individuals. The first decision to be made is: At what level will the quality assurance program be coordinated? By separating the collation, display, and dissemination of information from the analysis of problems, from the recommendation and taking of actions, and from the monitoring of problem-resolution activities, you can more easily decide who should participate in which activities.

Before delegating responsibility for certain activities, you should consider whether the activity would be best performed by an individual or a committee. Some functions can be handled better by an individual; for example, data management, technical advisory, and educational functions. Hospitals do not have to appoint a full-time coordinator to make use of all the data and resources available. This may be accomplished by a member of your management team.

Coordination by an Individual

Probably the greatest challenge to hospitals is using all the data that is routinely collected for various administrative and professional activities. Collating, displaying, and disseminating information can often be accomplished by one individual or coordinator on a part-time basis. This is particularly true in small hospitals. Minutes or other documentation of departmental and committee activities can be sent to the coordinator to be scanned for duplicative efforts. These data, and data from other sources, such as Professional Activity Survey (PAS) or PSRO can also be collated and disseminated by this individual to ascertain that appropriate committees or individuals receive and act upon the data.

The coordinator's duties can be expanded to include other responsibilities, such as analyzing data, providing educational and technical assistance to committees and departments in identifying and assessing problems, or recommending or monitoring actions. The scope of responsibilities and the person or group in the organization to whom the coordinator is functionally responsible (eg, chief executive officer, medical director, governing body, or director of medical education) will depend on the organizational level of the coordinator. Even if the role of the coordinator is expanded to include many coordinating activities, you should consider whether this is a full-time or a part-time position, whether it can be combined with other administrative responsibilities, and whether you want a staff or management official performing the function.

Another issue for consideration is whether this position should be filled by an individual currently on staff or by a new employee who is recruited from the outside. Many quality assurance experts recommend assigning the function to a current staff person who knows the institution and, consequently, is in a better position to facilitate change. The coordinator should have the respect of both the medical and professional staffs, possess skills in organization and communication, have an interest in quality assurance, be able to understand management objectives, and be able to implement a systems approach. Enhancing the credibility of the quality assurance program is far more important to establishing the program than possessing the required technical skills. Having expertise in quality assurance is an advantage, but it is not as important as the aforementioned characteristics. Furthermore, the right individual can be trained in quality assurance. The individual selected to assume the role can be a physician, nurse, social worker, or other health care professional.

Coordination by a medical director. After conducting an assessment of current quality assurance activities, one hospital decided that the full-time medical director was already functioning as the coordinator for many of the hospital's quality assurance activities. By formalizing this role and expanding activities in support service review and evaluation, the quality assurance activities throughout the hospital were integrated. (For an illustration of the reporting relationships and flow of information in this quality assurance program, see Figure 1, page 24.) His responsibilities for quality assurance include

- assisting committees and individuals in identifying known or perceived problems for study;
- setting priorities for the study of problems;
- reviewing action plans developed by the committee and departments;
- implementing actions approved by the medical staff executive committee or administration;
- monitoring problem resolution;
- communicating appropriate information from studies and data sources to other committees, departments, and persons affected by the study;
- managing the time and resources to conduct quality assurance activities that are integrated and not duplicative; and
- executing the *Memorandum of Understanding* between the hospital and the PSRO.

In this instance, the medical director's position is salaried and is accountable to the medical staff executive committee and the president of the hospital. One of the problems that can arise from such an arrangement, and one that should be carefully monitored, is the lack of interest in nonmedical staff problems. An advantage is that one official can take or delegate action.

If you currently have a salaried medical director, you might want to consider adopting this model; but if your medical director, chief of staff, or assistant chief of staff is an elected or part-time position, performing the coordination function might be too time-consuming.

Coordination by an assistant administrator. In another hospital, the assistant administrator already coordinated many of the medical staff quality assurance activities and assisted most of the support services in conducting reviews. After an initial assessment of the hospital's quality assurance activities, the assistant administrator was assigned full responsibility for implementing the quality assurance program throughout the hospital and was made accountable for the functions described in the previous example. Issues related to the medical staff were forwarded to the chief of staff for approval of actions, and the assistant administrator monitored resolution of the problems. Many of the identified problems related to the other professional staffs and departments can be resolved by the assistant administrator with other administrative staff and the department directors. (For an illustration of the reporting relationships and flow of information in this quality assurance program, see Figure 2, page 25.) The chief executive officer approved actions, was kept fully informed of professional staff activities, and intervened when necessary. As a member of the medical staff executive committee, the assistant administrator was aware of, and involved in, the resolution of medical staff problems.

In addition to those already described, the responsibilities of the assistant administrator include

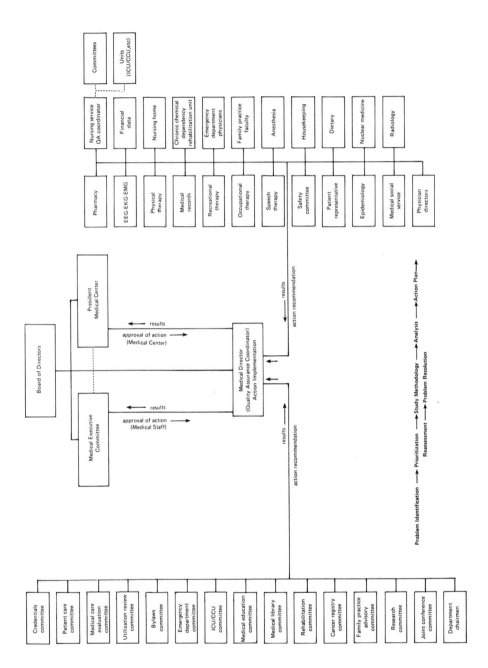

Figure 1. Illustration of the relationship be'tween the medical director or quality assurance coordinator and the medical committees and hospital departments and committees. Solid lines define the reporting relationship of quality assurance activities; arrows define flow of information.

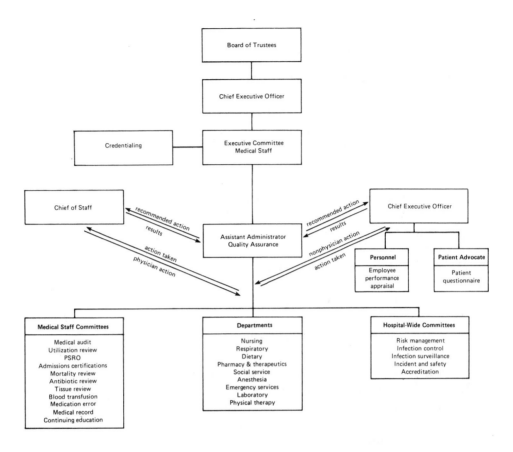

Figure 2. Illustration of the reporting lines and flow of information in a hospital where the assistant administrator coordinates quality assurance activities.

- facilitating the function of committees and departmental activities by providing data summaries;
- offering educational and technical assistance;
- managing data and information flow;
- coordinating "decentralized" activities of the medical staff, nursing, and support services;
- developing and modifying forms and systems;
- assisting committees in developing recommendations for actions and seeking approvals;
- alerting the chief executive officer and chief of staff to unresolved problems;
- coordinating follow-up on reports of external review agencies (ie, JCAH, PSRO, state licensing, etc);
- developing a centralized clearinghouse or library for quality assurance information;
- preparing summaries of information that will assist in identifying problems (ie, patient and staff surveys, complaint letters, etc); and
- preparing summary reports of quality assurance activities.

Coordination by One Committee

A committee can perform the coordinating function for hospital-wide quality assurance activities. In general, a quality assurance committee is responsible for reviewing identified problems and recommending further study or resolution of the problem, setting priorities for problem assessment, recommending action, and monitoring resolution of problems. It should be noted that it may be impractical for a quality assurance committee to identify problems, conduct studies, collate and disseminate information, and take actions. These tasks can best be completed within the departments or by individuals and committees involved in the evaluation of such aspects of care as blood utilization, intensive care, and antibiotic usage.

If your analysis of current activities revealed that one committee is involved in several quality assurance functions, consider whether this committee could coordinate all quality assurance activities. In some hospitals, a patient care committee serves as a forum for the discussion and resolution of problems and can easily assume responsibility for coordinating quality assurance activities.

We all know that committees can be ineffective, and it is difficult to hold a committee responsible for the coordination of the activities of other committees or departments. But there is great value in the multiple perspectives provided by members of a committee. The performance of a committee can be improved if its functions are clearly defined, if it receives appropriate and timely information, if its agendas are developed and adhered to, if group process techniques are used, if tasks are clearly assigned, if activities are completed on time, and if one individual is given responsibility for taking action or monitoring a specific problem.

The membership and reporting relationships of the quality assurance committee must be decided. The membership of the committee depends upon its role and functions. One hospital assigned responsibility for coordinating quality assurance activities and recommending actions to the utilization review committee. Membership includes representatives from each medical department, medical directors of the support services, and department directors. The audit, utilization review, and infection control coordinators are also members. The committee reports findings to the medical staff executive committee, which is responsible for credentialing and reports through the president to the governing body. To enhance communication, an assistant administrator, who is a member of the UR committee, is also a member of each medical staff committee. (For an illustration of the reporting relationships in this quality assurance program, see Figure 3 on the opposite page.)

If you are considering using the medical staff executive committee to coordinate quality assurance activities, several advantages and disadvantages should first be considered. On the positive side, this committee is already responsible for authorizing actions, and having it coordinate

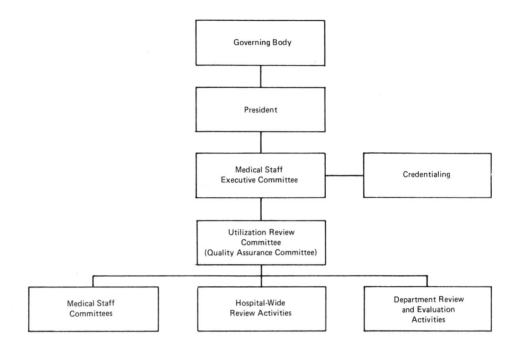

Figure 3. Illustration of reporting lines in a hospital in which one committee coordinates quality assurance activities.

quality assessment activities will preclude the need to establish another committee and possible creation of a power struggle. In addition, the medical staff committee already receives reports from committees, groups, and individual members of the medical staff. On the negative side, the committee might not be action-oriented or it might lack multidisciplinary input. Furthermore, it may already be so overburdened by the information it receives that patterns and problems would not be recognized. These points should be weighed carefully before deciding to coordinate activities through this committee.

Regardless of the committee's organizational level, members must be particularly sensitive to political and personal relationships, and they must respect the confidentiality of the information they review. If one committee is to coordinate quality assurance activities, you must decide whether or not committee membership will rotate. In part, this will depend upon the organizational level of the committee and its functions. Several hospitals altered the level of membership of the quality assurance committee after a few meetings. For example, one hospital had established a quality assurance committee at a departmental level, but later upgraded the organizational level of the committee to enhance the protection accorded to confidentiality of information. Another hospital established a quality assurance committee at the same organizational level as the medical staff executive committee. Six months later the reporting relationship was modified so that the quality assurance committee reported to the medical staff executive committee. A common arrangement is to have a quality assurance committee that reports to the medical staff executive committee and the chief executive officer, and that is comprised of the director of nursing, chairpersons of several key medical staff committees, assistant administrators, and other management staff. In several hospitals this committee identifies problems and assigns problem assessment to task force groups or study committees for further investigation.

Coordination by Several Quality Assurance Committees

If you decide to coordinate activities by a committee, the scope of the committee's activities should be defined. Although there are many advantages to having a multidisciplinary committee, it may be necessary or desirable to separate the coordination of medical staff activities from those of other professional staffs. If this is the case, you must decide how the activities of the other professionals will be coordinated. How will problems that involve more than one discipline be solved? How will activities be integrated? And finally, how will priorities be set to assure equitability?

Some hospitals have established two committees to coordinate quality assurance activities. One committee, the medical staff quality assurance committee, is responsible for coordination of medical staff functions and is comprised of the chairpersons of the medical audit, utilization review, infection control, blood utilization and surgical case review, safety, pharmacy and therapeutics, and emergency services committees. Another possible approach is to have medical staff department chairpersons comprise the committee. The chairperson of the executive committee chairs the medical staff quality assurance committee. The other committee, the professional staff quality assurance committee, is comprised of the director of nursing, and the department heads of pharmacy, social service, dietary, respiratory, and physical therapy. A member of the medical staff quality assurance committee and the assistant administrator for medical staff affairs also serve on the professional staff quality assurance committee.

This two-committee arrangement may be desirable if your hospital is large and conducts many evaluation activities, if your medical staff is reluctant to share information with other staffs, or if one committee would be too large to be effective. Other members that should be included either full-time or on an ad-hoc basis are the directors of nuclear medicine, the laboratory, radiology, and anesthesiology. The two-committee model can also serve as an interim approach until it is feasible to form one committee. (For an illustration of the reporting relationships in this quality assurance program, see Figure 4 on the opposite page.)

Whether your organization includes one or two committees, the responsibilities generally assigned to a quality assurance committee include

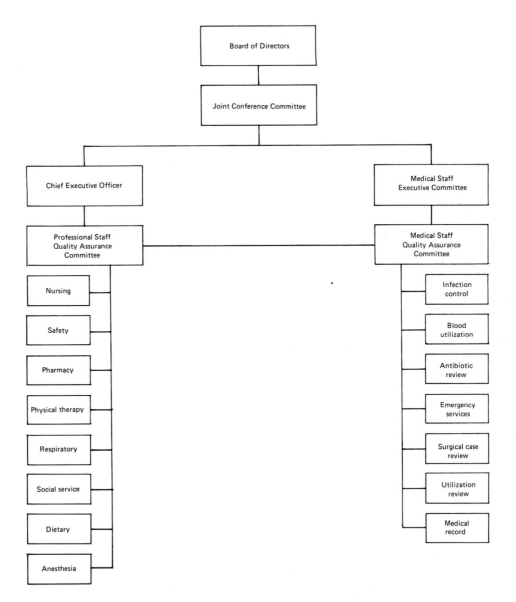

Figure 4. Illustration of the reporting relationships in a hospital in which more than one committee has responsibility for coordination of quality assurance activities.

- synthesizing problem data from multiple sources;
- reviewing the reports and minutes of committees, departments, and individuals;
- reviewing problems that are likely to have an impact on the quality of care or on service rendered to patients;
- directing appropriate committees and individuals to conduct further investigation of specific topics and to monitor corrective action to sustain problem resolution;
- providing feedback to committees and individuals involved in quality assurance;
- establishing or recommending priorities for study of problems or problem resolution;
- reporting committee findings and results;
- conducting an annual evaluation of the quality assurance program;
- directing action for problem resolution (or assuring that this is appropriately delegated); and
- monitoring resolution of problems.

Depending on its composition, the quality assurance committee may also approve action and assume a risk management function as well.

Coordination by a Quality Assurance Department

Another option that several hospitals have chosen is to coordinate the quality assurance activities of the various departments and committees through a quality assurance department. In most instances, the department is composed of individuals already involved in quality assurance, such as the utilization review coordinator, nursing and medical audit coordinators, and the infection control nurse. However, you should also consider including the patient representative, discharge planner, data retriever or data abstractor, and other individuals not usually considered within the scope of quality assurance activities, such as the tumor registrar or blood bank statistician. Quality assurance departments can vary in size. A teaching hospital with over 1,000 beds set up its department to include seven full-time staff and a director. (For an illustration of the reporting relationships in this quality assurance program, see Figure 5 on the opposite page.)

The quality assurance department usually serves as a clearinghouse for all quality assurance information; it does not serve as a decision-making body. Staff provide technical assistance in problem identification and assessment, and prepare quality assurance activity reports for the governing body, administration, and medical staff executive committee. The advantages to this arrangement are that department staff are cross-trained, information is centralized, duplication of staff and committee efforts are minimized, and roles are more clearly delineated.

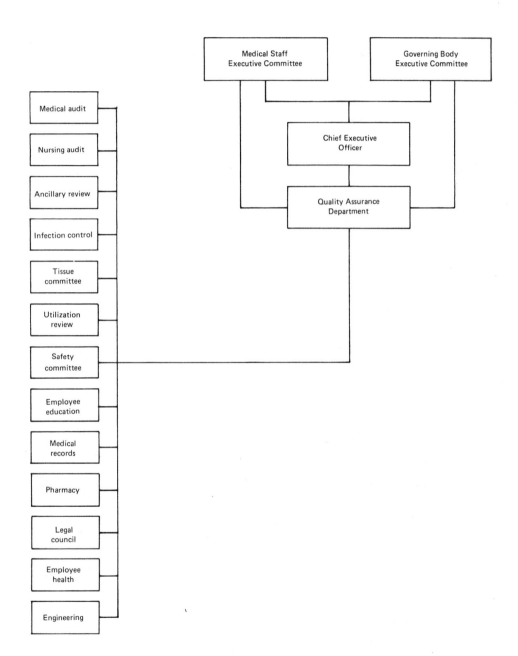

Figure 5. Illustration of reporting lines in a hospital in which quality assurance activities are coordinated by a quality assurance department.

The department director can be a physician, nurse, or administrator. Depending on the qualifications of the director and the size of the department, the director and staff may serve on various quality assurance committees, or they may actually perform committee functions. This may be most practical for utilization review and infection control monitoring. If your assessment of current activities identified several individuals involved in multiple quality assurance activities, consider whether or not a departmental approach would be feasible. When considering staffing of a quality assurance department, consider what activities necessitate full-time staff and what activities can be performed on a part-time basis. For example, if the utilization review function is satisfactorily performed on a part-time basis or if converting to a focused review process has created free time for the utilization review coordinator, consider what additional functions or tasks this individual can undertake. Other activities that can be incorporated within, or be closely related to, the quality assurance department are the risk management activity and hospital-wide education activities.

Coordination by Combined Approaches

In many hospitals, the most effective way to coordinate quality assurance activities is to use a combined approach. A workable approach utilizes a quality assurance committee and an individual, or a committee and a department. Another approach is to have separate quality assurance committees for the professional and medical staffs, and a quality assurance department to coordinate the activities of both committees. (For illustrations of the reporting relationships and flow of information in quality assurance programs using these two approaches, see Figures 6 and 7 on the opposite page.)

A combined approach is usually necessary when one or more committees will coordinate quality assurance activities, because it is difficult for one committee to adequately manage data and activities. A combined approach is also advisable when the quality assurance committee has decision-making responsibilities, such as when quality assurance activities are coordinated by the medical staff executive committee. In a combined approach, the individual or department serves as a support unit to the committee or group. Generally, they perform the functions that are difficult for a committee to perform, such as

- managing data and, to some extent, protecting confidentiality;
- providing educational support, including technical assistance;
- investigating problems;
- assuring comprehensiveness; and
- assigning others to conduct studies.

Another factor to be considered is that individuals or departments are held accountable; this is often not the case with a committee.

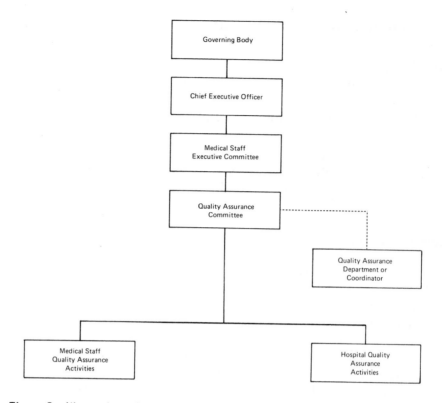

Figure 6. Illustration of reporting lines in hospitals in which activities are coordinated by one quality assurance committee and a quality assurance department or coordinator.

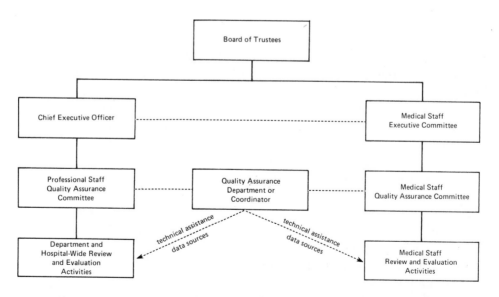

Figure 7. Illustration of reporting lines and flow of information in a hospital in which quality assurance activities are coordinated by two or more hospital quality assurance committees and a quality assurance department or coordinator.

Consolidating Review and Evaluation Activities

Once the decision regarding how to coordinate hospital-wide quality assurance activities has been made, consider consolidating some of your committees. Consolidation of activities can result in benefits to committee members by making meetings more productive and by requiring considerably less of their time. These benefits can help "sell" the idea of quality assurance integration. The activities of the medical and nursing staffs, especially in large hospitals, can be coordinated and consolidated separately, and then integrated into the hospital-wide quality assurance program.

Medical Staff Quality Assurance Activities

Medical staff monitoring activities are usually performed by committees that are isolated from one another. As mentioned earlier, the functions must be performed, but they do not have to be performed by a committee. Your assessment of current activities may indicate that certain committees have similar memberships. Or, the assessment may indicate several committees performing related or duplicative functions. Often this happens because committee roles are not clearly delineated, little communication exists between committees or medical staff departments in a departmentalized organization, or overall direction is lacking. The medical staff must support consolidation and reorganize their activities.

One hospital's medical staff elected to consolidate the activities of eleven committees into three: quality assurance, systems and procedures, and education (see Figure 8 on the opposite page). The library and education committees were organized into the education committee, and the emergency room, laboratory and safety, and disaster committees became the systems and procedures committee. The quality assurance committee encompassed the activities of the following six committees: infection control, medical audit, medical records, utilization review, pharmacy and therapeutics, and blood and tissue. (Note: The quality assurance committee is, in effect, the infection control committee and the systems and procedures committee is the safety committee which are required by JCAH standards.) The chairpersons of each committee sit on, and report to, the medical staff executive committee, which also performs the credentialing function. The hospital administrator and the hospital president are members of the executive committee and act on relevant information or communicate it to the professional staff and governing body. This arrangement dramatically reduced the amount of time required for meetings and significantly increased committee productivity and communication.

Another arrangement is to have one committee that is responsible for monitoring activities, including blood utilization, tissue review, medi-

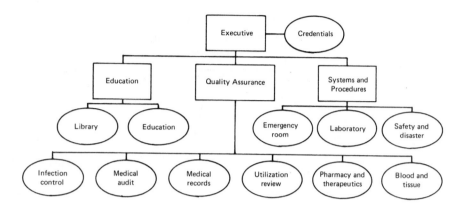

Figure 8. Committee structure was reorganized so that the functions of six previously existing committees are now handled by the quality assurance committee; the functions of two former committees, by the education committee; and the functions of three former committees, by the systems and procedures committee. The chairmen of the three newly organized committees sit on the executive committee and, thus, report to it and to each other. The boxes represent committees; the circles represent specific functions of those committees. The horizontal lines indicate communication channels among the various functions and committees; the vertical lines show both communication and reporting channels.

From Dietz JW, Phillips JL: The quality assurance committee in the hospital structure. *QRB* 6:8-12, Jan 1980, p 11. Reprinted with permission.

cal record review, and antibiotic review; a utilization review committee; and a medical audit committee that studies problems identified from the monitoring or utilization review committees. Regular reports are made to a medical director who coordinates the information and reports items requiring action approval to the medical staff executive committee, which also is responsible for credentialing. Issues related to education are sent to the director of medical education for resolution.

Nursing Service Quality Assurance Activities

The evaluation activities of a nursing department can be coordinated separately, and then integrated into the hospital-wide quality assurance program. This may be an effective method in large hospitals. Nursing services should be evaluated at least quarterly. What review activities will be conducted, how often, and by whom are issues that cross departments, units, and special care areas.

The nursing service at one hospital centralized its nursing evaluation activities (see Figure 9, page 36). Through the director of nursing, evaluation activities were linked to education efforts, to performance appraisals, to changes in policies and procedures, and to other manage-

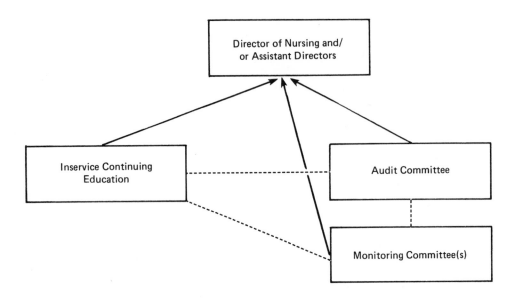

Figure 9. Solid lines illustrate reporting lines and dotted lines illustrate flow of information in a hospital in which nursing review and evaluation activities were consolidated. The director of nursing is a member of the hospital quality assurance committee.

ment decisions. The nursing evaluation activities were conducted by a nursing audit committee and two monitoring committees. One monitoring committee reviewed blood administration, IV therapy, and isolation. The other monitoring committee reviewed cardiopulmonary resuscitation, medication incidents, and any special problems. For example, a problem of increased incidence of decubiti was identified by the nursing audit committee. Corrective action was taken and the second monitoring committee followed the problem until the incident rate had decreased to an acceptable level.

Comment

The assessment of current activities may indicate that you can improve the effectiveness of various functions and increase communication by consolidating and coordinating departmental activities. If this is the case, management must be fully involved and must support the activity, and staff must be informed when decisions are made.

Chapter 5. Implementing a Quality Assurance Program

After analyzing your current quality assurance program, you must determine how much change is necessary to correct any inadequacies or inefficiencies in the program. If, for example, you find that most activities are performed satisfactorily, but that they are not sufficiently coordinated or integrated, you may only have to make a few minor changes. If, on the other hand, you find that few activities are performed satisfactorily, that activities are not coordinated or integrated at all, that no follow-up is conducted after corrective action has been taken, that real problems are often not addressed, or that many problems reported to the medical staff executive committee are not resolved, you may wish to make major changes in the quality assurance program.

Once you have identified activities that have to be improved and determined how much change is necessary to improve them, you must then determine how much change you can bring about successfully. This will depend upon the number of inefficiencies that you have identified, the time and effort required to correct them, and the "climate" for change within your hospital. These considerations are preliminary but crucial to the development of a workable quality assurance program, as well as to the transition period between development of the plan and full implementation of the program.

Among the first things you must do in attempting to implement a successful quality assurance program are to develop a written plan, identify needed change, secure staff approval and support of the program, facilitate the program's success, and plan how you are going to phase in the new quality assurance program. The period of transition between development of the plan and full implementation of the program is critical to the program's success.

Developing a Quality Assurance Plan

Whether you are undertaking minor or major changes in your hospital, you must remember that oftentimes problems are finally solved only after many methods have been tried to solve them. Consequently, you should regard your quality assurance plan as a working document that is subject to continuous change based on the degree of success or failure you experience in conducting everyday quality assurance activities. Although the goal or purpose of the plan will most likely remain unchanged, the methods or objectives that are used to achieve that purpose may change constantly. With this in mind, you can begin to develop your quality assurance plan.

A hospital's quality assurance plan should present a clear picture of the quality assurance program so that the program can be easily understood by both staff and external reviewers. This can usually be accomplished by a brief description of the program and a copy of the program's organizational chart. It is important to emphasize that the description does not have to be lengthy, and the plan does not have to contain copies of documents that are located elsewhere in the hospital. The plan can simply reference these documents if necessary.

There are five elements that you can include in your plan that will help to illustrate the program. These elements are a statement of the purpose of the program; a statement of the scope of the program; a description of how the program will be administered and coordinated; a description of how the hospital intends to use a problem-focused approach to assess quality of care; and a description of the evaluation mechanisms of the program. (See Appendix A for examples of quality assurance plans developed by five hospitals of various sizes that are located in different parts of the country.)

Statement of purpose. Although you need not necessarily state the purpose of the quality assurance program in the plan, it is helpful to do so. The statement will remind staff of their goal and will guide them in evaluating and, if necessary, changing activities to achieve the goal. If you include a statement of purpose, it should be clear and concise, and it should include the goals and objectives you have set for the program.

Statement of scope. The scope of the program should be described briefly and illustrated in an organizational chart. The chart will also serve to illustrate responsibility for quality assurance activities. It is important to note that the plan should include the quality assurance activities of all disciplines involved in patient care, not just those of the medical and nursing staffs.

Administration and coordination. The means by which you will administer and coordinate quality assurance activities should be described in the plan. Although the organizational chart will depict reporting relationships, you might wish to include a description of the functions of the committee, group, individual, and/or department responsible for administration and coordination.

Problem-focused approach. The five components of a quality assurance program that are identified in the hospital quality assurance standard include the following:

- the identification of important problems;
- objective assessment of the cause and scope of problems, including the determination of priorities;
- implementation of actions designed to correct problems;
- monitoring activities designed to assure that the desired results have been achieved and sustained; and
- documentation that reasonably substantiates the effectiveness of the overall program.

Because these five components are considered integral to an effective quality assurance program, they will be considered as a whole during an accreditation survey. The plan should therefore specify what mechanisms the hospital will use to identify problems, who sets priorities, who is responsible for assessing problems and monitoring resolution, and who approves and/or takes action.

Evaluation mechanism. The last element that should be included in a quality assurance plan is a description of how the program will be evaluated (see Chapter 11). A statement of who will conduct the evaluation may also be included.

Identifying Needed Change

The climate for change within your hospital will influence the amount of change you can effect. Although altering the responsibilities or reporting relationships of a committee or dissolving a committee altogether may be desirable from an organizational perspective, it might be impractical because of the attitudes or "clout" of committee members. Strong resistance to change can seriously hinder overall efforts to implement an effective program. Unless the incentive for change comes from the group that needs change or from key leaders in the organization, and unless all individuals involved in the change actively support it, efforts to organize for change will be difficult. In fact, staff motivation can be one of the most difficult problems to solve. Because negative attitudes can thwart efforts to change, quality assurance planners must confront them openly and honestly, and they must try to prevent the spread of any rumors that distort people's views of the quality assurance program.

To identify the necessary changes, determine first the strengths and weaknesses of current activities. The use of a systems approach and force field analysis techniques will help you identify the strengths and weaknesses of current activities; develop a plan to correct weaknesses while maintaining strengths; designate a time frame for implementation of the program; and specify the individual or group responsible for implementing the quality assurance program. When you begin to plan for change, compare your quality assurance plan to the assessment of your current activities. Questions 1 through 3 in Chapter 2 relate to the scope and comprehensiveness of the program, questions 2 and 9 cover administration and coordination, questions 4 through 8 relate to the organization and use of a problem-focused approach, and question 10 concerns evaluation of the program and functions. By using this method and the more formal methods mentioned in Chapter 2, you will be able to determine the impact of the program throughout the organization, and you can plan activities that will facilitate acceptance of the program and achievement of its goals and objectives.

Securing Staff Approval and Support

If there is a single factor underlying the success of a quality assurance program it is the type and level of staff involvement in program activities. However, staff frequently express concern that many professionals lack the interest and motivation to participate in, or cooperate with, hospital quality assurance activities. Our work in hospitals has taught us that, regardless of the form it takes, resistance to quality assurance is most often rooted in lack of familiarity with its purpose and process. In addition, because of their genuine and considerable efforts to provide excellent care and evaluate the quality of that care, staff frequently resent the time-consuming (and costly) requirements for quality assurance activity that are imposed by outside organizations. To successfully implement a quality assurance program, it is important to identify areas needing change and to consider the factors that will facilitate the program's success.

Facilitating the Program's Success

Before developing a specific approach to staff motivation, consider the following factors: the structure and environment of, and climate for change within, the hospital; the extent and type of resistance; the extent and type of support; the strengths and weaknesses of the current program; and the type of actions required to facilitate staff participation and/or support. A review of these factors will help you to focus on the strengths in the system and target actions to correct specific weaknesses.

   The support of the governing body, administration, and key physicians. Determine how actively and positively the governing body, administration, and influential physicians support the concept of quality assurance. The greater the level of support from key decision-makers, the more direct and effective you can be in securing staff support of and participation in quality assurance activities. In situations where high-level support is lacking, more informal or individualized approaches to facilitating participation may be necessary.

The organizational hierarchy. Staff participation can be secured successfully only if those who have the authority to elicit responsive behavior from uncooperative and resistant professionals support the program and if those who are responsible for assuring responsive behavior implement the program. Those responsible for implementing a quality assurance program should have positions in the organizational hierarchy that ensure the required authority and responsibility. Lines of authority and responsibility should be delineated clearly.

The knowledge and place in the organizational hierarchy of those with authority and responsibility for the overall quality assurance program. Staff participation and support can be secured more readily when those responsible for the quality assurance program are knowledgeable about quality assurance and hold key positions in the organization. If those in key positions are not knowledgeable, their education should be of primary importance.

The interpersonal and teaching skills of those responsible for implementing the quality assurance program. Whether actions to facilitate participation are conducted on a group or on an informal, person-to-person basis, those responsible for these actions should have strong interpersonal and teaching skills.

Staff resistance. A few isolated people from any professional group can disrupt a quality assurance program; entire groups of professionals within an institution can actively resist the development of a sound, effective program. The actions selected to secure staff participation depend on how many resist the quality assurance activity, how strongly they resist it, and how influential they are in the facility.

The personalities of those who resist. An understanding of the personalities of those who resist will determine the type of encouragement that will be most effective. For example, one might consider whether low-key or high-pressure "salesmen" are likely to be effective with a particular professional or professional group. Once the approach is determined, select the salesman appropriate to the need.

Use of quality assurance findings. Staff motivation is increased when confidentiality is maintained and when tangible evidence of the impact of quality assurance can be demonstrated. Even highly motivated, cooperative staff will resist change when negative quality assurance findings are not handled properly or when the impact of quality assurance activities cannot be seen.

The extent of outside pressure for involvement in quality assurance. When pressure from outside sources (eg, local PSRO, insurance companies, other third-party payers, or regulatory agencies) is substantial, demonstrating how professional goals are served by cooperation and involvement in quality assurance activities can enhance staff motivation.

Planning the Transition Period

Because immediate implementation of the entire quality assurance program is unlikely, you should plan to phase in the program. The success of the program may depend on how carefully you plan the transition period. Although it may be necessary to conduct educational efforts and to change roles, responsibilities, policies, and procedures, the sequence and timing of implementing these activities may be critical to success. Consequently, organize this period carefully and, in the transition plan, specifically identify the activity and the individual responsible, the individuals affected, and the time frame for implementation. (Although there are a variety of resources that will help you in the transition period, the following two may be of particular interest: *Organizational Transitions, Managing Complex Change** and *The Manager's Guide to Change.*†)

You may want to assign the responsibility for implementing the plan to one person. For example, an assistant administrator, a medical director, or a quality assurance coordinator could be assigned responsibility for managing transition activities. You could also select someone who is not currently involved in quality assurance activities. Whoever you select should have authority to implement change and should be respected by administrative, professional, and support staffs. The assignment can be temporary, lasting only until the quality assurance program is fully implemented or it can be a permanent quality assurance related responsibility.

In planning your transition strategy, be sure to identify all individuals involved in the changes and to consider the effect of proposed changes on them. Will they resist change, accept it, or be indifferent? Will they be threatened by it? Even though people may complain about their work, they are often reluctant to relinquish responsibility for it, and they resent having that responsibility taken from them. How the change is perceived by the affected individuals and how it affects their jobs is important and should be considered in planning the transition strategy. The type and amount of change also should be considered. For example, if your transition strategy calls for a training program on how to conduct problem-focused studies, you should consider how much training is needed, what kind of training is needed, and who needs it. An individual trained in traditional medical audit may be less adaptable to new methods than an individual who has little or no training in evaluation. Each of these individuals may require different types and amounts of training.

The transition plan should include time frames for implementation of each activity. This encourages a gradual approach to change. For example, if the quality assurance plan requires that a department coordinate

---

*Beckhard R, Harris RT: *Organizational Transitions: Managing Complex Change.* Reading, Mass: Addison-Wesley Publishing Co, 1977.
†Burack H, Torda F: *The Manager's Guide to Change.* Belmont, Calif: A Lifetime Learning Publication, 1979.

activities, you may establish a timetable for gradually reassigning or hiring staff. Likewise, if the plan calls for combining or eliminating several committees, you can establish a timetable for accomplishing this gradually.

Strategies for Change

There are numerous ways to achieve change. Because each hospital is unique, no single "correct" action will serve to motivate all staff. The following are some of the more general ways that, regardless of the amount of change that has to be made, may help you through the transition period. (For a discussion of the change strategies that can be used to correct problems in patient care and clinical performance, see Chapter 9.)

Involve all key individuals in establishing the quality assurance program or in implementing a specific quality assurance activity. Several hospitals have found that including key members of the medical staff— even those most resistant to quality assurance—in the planning stages is a successful strategy for change. They have identified the two or three most influential medical staff members in the hospital and involved them in planning, organizing, and implementing the quality assurance program. If such leaders cannot be actively involved in the process of change itself, they can facilitate change by giving the program their support. Individuals involved in the planning and implementation process have an investment in the success of the quality assurance program and will support change. When key individuals are not involved in or do not actively support the quality assurance program, hospital staff could perceive the program as unimportant. Consequently, hospital staff will be less likely to attach high priority to their own involvement in the program.

Promote the quality assurance program. Develop a campaign to promote the quality assurance program. Staff are more likely to accept the program if they are kept informed. Let staff know what changes are being made and how the changes will benefit the organization. Keep them informed of their role in the program. The quality assurance program will be more successful if you present it as an important priority that everyone has some responsibility for and involvement in. This approach will emphasize the program's permanence, and staff will be less likely to withhold their support because they consider it a fad.

Use formal and informal lines of communication. In attempting to secure staff support and participation, both formal and informal lines of communication in the hospital should be used and used appropriately. Formal communications (eg, memoranda and inservice programs) from administration or department heads and publicity about the program are most likely to be effective when addressed to large groups of people. Formal communications should therefore be used when it is necessary to motivate a large number of staff members.

Informal communication (eg, discussions over coffee) work best when a limited number of people are involved, particularly those who are resistant and need additional knowledge about the purpose and process of quality assurance. Both formal and informal communications are likely to be most effective when provided by individuals who are perceived as having influence in the hospital.

Develop an appropriate mix of confidentiality and openness. An open and positive attitude toward the quality assurance program will encourage communication, support, and participation. Staff are more likely to be involved in quality assurance activities when the quality assurance program receives wide publicity, when activities are not shrouded in secrecy, and when all but the most sensitive quality assurance related meetings are open to interested staff. Such openness discourages suspicion and anxiety about the quality assurance program or its components.

Conduct general education programs. Change is facilitated when staff know and understand the requirements for review and evaluation, particularly within their own disciplines. Because of this, orientation and other education programs should be conducted within each service and various methods should be used to maintain regular communication. These efforts will help staff understand the need for an integrated quality assurance program, dispel doubts about the value of the program, and help ensure that the changes are not seen as threatening.

Conduct specific education programs. Staff and committee members who are directly involved in quality assurance might require specific training in the performance and coordination of review and evaluation activities. Many resources that can be used for this training already exist within hospitals. These include staff who have previous experience in review and evaluation; journals and other literature on quality assurance, problem identification, and criteria development; and inservice education seminars. Such resources should be evaluated carefully before a decision is made to utilize outside resources.

Ask friends and peers to help. Ask friends or respected peers of resistant staff to explain the purpose and usefulness of particular quality assurance activities and to encourage participation by such staff.

Focus committee and staff activities. Regardless of how many changes you intend to make in your current quality assurance program, you should immediately begin to focus on problems in patient care. Initially, staff should be encouraged to focus on known problems in patient care that are simple to study, that require use of few criteria, and that are resolvable. The support and interest of staff who have resisted the program can be obtained if they see old problems actually being solved. Also, other staff and members of quality assurance committees will be encouraged, and their interest and participation in the program will increase.

Select problem areas of interest and concern to resistant staff. Even if these problems do not otherwise have a high priority, it might be useful to select a few of them for study. Resolution of such problems might capture the attention of uninvolved or uninterested staff and provide a positive introduction to, or experience with, quality assurance activity.

Involve influential but resistant staff on quality assurance committees in areas of particular interest to them. This provides them with a positive experience and increases their emotional commitment to, as well as cognitive understanding of, quality assurance activity.

Change committee or individual functions. It might not be feasible to change staff reporting relationships during the first phase of program implementation. It might be more practical to share information regarding findings and activities among staff and use such information to justify changes you wish to make later. Such changes will be more acceptable as committee members become more comfortable with the program and more knowledgeable about their tasks, and as staff begin to accept and respect the roles of the committees in implementing change.

Provide adequate resource support. All quality assurance activities must have adequate resource support so that staff time is focused on issues of professional concern rather than routine support functions.

Document the operations and progress of the program. Although the quality assurance standard does not require hospitals to develop policies and procedures for quality assurance activities, such policies and procedures are useful in implementing a quality assurance program. Written policies and procedures clarify the purpose of the program and the roles, responsibilities, and reporting relationships of the committees, departments, and/or individuals who participate in the program. Policies and procedures can also guide staff in planning, implementing, and evaluating the program. Hospital and medical staff bylaws may need to be revised once you are satisfied that the quality assurance program is effective and efficient.

Formalize the quality assurance program. Policies and procedures and bylaws will assist in defining and formalizing the quality assurance program. However, additional tasks such as developing a budget for the quality assurance program and writing job descriptions for staff may be desirable.

Comment

Those who are responsible for implementing quality assurance programs should understand that it will be difficult to obtain the active support and participation of all staff. Despite careful and vigorous efforts to secure staff participation, some individuals may remain suspicious, anxious, uncooperative, or uninterested in quality assurance activities.

However, even though opposition may make it more difficult, you *can* design an effective, efficient quality assurance program. Early implementation of some of the practical actions outlined in this chapter should help minimize resistance to change. The time invested in planning for change and in carefully conducting and evaluating each activity will result in an effective program that most staff will accept.

Chapter 6. Identifying Problems

Although the quality assurance standard of the Joint Commission on Accreditation of Hospitals emphasizes the identification and resolution of known or suspected problems in patient care, the hospital and medical staffs' responsibility for identifying and resolving problems is not new. Professional and ethical responsibility to provide care of high quality has always been inherent in the practice of health care, and problems in delivery of that care should be addressed and resolved. The potential for improvement in the delivery of care should be recognized when it exists. When the improvement is likely to have significant impact on patient care, it should be addressed quickly. Toward this end, hospital quality assurance programs should be designed to synthesize data collected from each quality assurance activity and from other internal and external data sources, to identify problems that are suggested by the data, and to resolve the problems in reasonable order of priority.

This chapter defines the general characteristics of problems that require assessment; describes the use of multiple data sources and identifies internal and external data sources for problem identification; illustrates problem indicators that can be employed in analyzing the data; describes elements that should be included in documentation of problem identification; and discusses how to organize the problem identification activity.

Problem identification can be accomplished efficiently, effectively, and economically when multiple data sources are used and interpreted carefully, and when the organization of problem identification activities suits the unique structure of the hospital. If you consider information from as many internal and external data sources as possible and display the information clearly and logically, it is more likely that you will identify high impact problems in care. If topics are selected only on the basis of individual practitioner interest, if such topics are restricted to an area of care that involves only a small number of patients, or if there is little likelihood of change, you might overlook the opportunity to investigate problems of broader import. Because topic selection based on individual practitioner interest often results in ineffective and inefficient use of quality assurance resources, areas of care that represent small patient, provider, or problem (diagnosis or procedure) populations should be evaluated only if a problem is suspected.

You also might miss the opportunity to identify important problems if topics are selected on a rotating service basis only. For example, is pediatric gastroenteritis studied for no reason other than that the pediatric service must conduct a study? If no problems exist in the admission, diagnosis, treatment, or discharge of children with this diagnosis, there is no need for a full-scale assessment. Such an assessment should be conducted only when a problem is suspected.

Use of multiple data sources increases the likelihood that major problems will be identified. One could argue that a committee of physicians and nurses should "know" existing problems. Often they do; however, important problems can be lost or ignored if one relies on intuition and observation without supporting information.

General Characteristics of Problems Needing Assessment

A problem can be defined as a deviation from an expected occurrence that cannot be justified as appropriate under the given circumstances. (For example, a high rate of repeated radiologic studies that occurs because of improper or ineffective patient preparation is neither an expected result of the diagnostic procedure nor one that can be readily justified.) Problems that could be selected as the focus of a quality assurance activity have the characteristics that are described under the next two headings.

Resolvable Problems

Because the goal of quality assurance activity is improved patient care and outcome, it is sensible to concentrate efforts in areas where significant improvement is likely to occur and to focus attention on problems that appear to be resolvable. For example, it is not possible to prevent all mortality associated with myocardial infarction. Similarly, some medication errors will occur despite the intensity of quality assurance activities. Thus, if you have a choice between problems to address, first pursue those for which the potential for improvement in patient care or outcomes appears to be the greatest.

Positive Impact on Patient Care and Outcomes

Documentation of high quality care may occur as a serendipitous effect of problem-focused assessments. However, it should occur primarily as part of a reevaluation that demonstrates problem resolution. Focusing the quality assurance program on problems whose resolution is expected to have an important, positive impact on patient care and outcome is critical to reasonable allocation of scarce quality assurance resources.

Use of Multiple Data Sources

The use of multiple data sources helps assure that major problem areas are identified regardless of the source of the problem (eg, an individual, service, department, or unit) and that problems which have a high impact on patient care are identified rather than only those that will be convenient to assess. When multiple data sources are used, it is likely that more important problems will be identified. Although examples of internal and external data sources are provided in the quality assurance standard and in this *Guide,* the provision of examples is not intended to imply that the use of specific sources, or the use of all listed sources, is required. A hospital should consider all available data sources and select those which will be most applicable to its own needs.

Data sources classified as internal are those generated in the hospital, such as incident reports, infection surveillance reports, and tissue review. External data sources are those generated by organizations outside the hospital. Internal data sources are more familiar and, currently, are more likely to be used in quality assurance activities. However, the importance of external data in problem identification is increasing.

Examples of internal data sources include, but are not limited to,

- medical records,
- incident reports,
- infection control reports,
- blood utilization reports,
- pharmacy reports,
- laboratory reports,
- committee/department reports,
- generic screening criteria,
- patient bills,
- staff research and evaluation reports,
- staff surveys,
- patient surveys,
- direct observation, and
- credentialing reports.

Examples that illustrate the use of internal data sources are provided at the end of this chapter. Information from many of these sources is usually generated routinely.

External data sources are used by hospitals less frequently. However, their use should be seriously considered. As external agencies (eg, PSROs, cost review commissions, and third-party payers) become more effective in data collection, the data they generate will play a more important role in hospital quality assurance activities. Also, health care literature, although not necessarily hospital-specific, can be used as a reference or comparison point for identification of hospital problems. Examples of external data sources include, but are not limited to,

- PSRO reports,
- HSA reports,
- PAS reports,
- Hospital Activity Survey (HAS) reports,
- cost review commission reports,
- third-party payer reports, and
- literature related to health care.

Examples that illustrate the use of external data sources are also provided at the end of this chapter. Data are being generated by these sources with greater frequency and, in some cases (eg, PSROs), such data can be specifically requested by an individual hospital.

Interpretation of Data Sources

To use multiple data sources for problem identification, it is necessary to extract the most relevant data. Data can be displayed, reviewed, analyzed, and interpreted in numerous ways. For purposes of problem identification, presentation of data should be simple, straightforward, and logical. Once data are logically organized and displayed, it is then possible to look for several problem indicators, such as

- single events of major impact (eg, malfunction of vital equipment);
- recurrent problems that collectively are of concern (eg, moderately large numbers of rescheduled radiologic diagnostic procedures or specific types of medication errors);
- trends that give reason for concern (eg, increase in a disease-specific mortality rate, nosocomial infection rate, or occurrence of decubiti on a specific service); and
- issues raised by multiple sources (eg, incidence of unjustified hospitalization for dilatation and curettage noted by utilization review committee, local PSRO, and third-party payer).

When interpreting data that suggest the presence of a problem, consider the description, implications, and potential explanations of the problem as defined below.

Descriptions. Measures of extent and site of problem, including frequency (eg, how many), topic (eg, single unit transfusions), occurrence in specified period of time (eg, number of events in the last six months), amount of change over time (eg, a 20% increase from the third to fourth quarters of this year), and place of occurrence (eg, unit or service).

Implications of the extent of the problem. This includes patient outcomes that might occur if the problem were to remain unsolved (eg, increased mortality, increased complications, or potentially compensable events).

Potential explanations of why the problem exists. That is, what are possible reasons for the deviation from the expected event that is observed in the data?

Documentation of Problem Identification

Although the quality assurance standard does not require a specific format for documentation of problem identification, any description of identified problems might include a brief statement on each of the following points:

- known or suspected problems or areas amenable to improvement;
- any data source or criteria used to identify known or suspected problems;
- summary of probable extent of problem area (eg, 30% mortality for acute myocardial infarction; 40% normal pathology reports after appendectomy);
- rough estimates of the anticipated health benefits (eg, reduced exposure to radiation, reduced risk of patient falls); and
- possible explanations of the problems (eg, inappropriate prescribing habits, delayed reporting of stat laboratory results, excessive waiting time in emergency room, poor staffing patterns, knowledge or skill deficiencies).

Example of Documentation of Problem Identification

The following is an example of documentation of problem identification. The intensive care nursery (ICN) and respiratory therapy department of a 428-bed community hospital became concerned about changes in oxygen therapy that were occurring without written orders.*

A. *Suspected problem.* Changes in oxygen concentration or discontinuation of oxygen for infants in the ICN are being instituted without written orders from the responsible pediatrician.
B. *Data source and criteria.* The suspected problem was discussed at a nursing staff meeting. The relevant criterion is the hospital's policy that oxygen therapy may not be discontinued or altered without a written physician order.
C. *Probable extent of problem.* Insufficient data available to estimate extent.

---

*Adapted with the permission of June Sullivan, assistant director, Medical Records, and Tom Woolbright, director of respiratory therapy, Forrest General Hospital, Hattiesburg, Miss.

D. *Anticipated benefit.* Elimination of the confusion caused by lack of written orders should result in reduction of the medical, legal, and economic risks associated with inappropriate use of oxygen.

E. *Possible explanation of the problem.* Possible causes include pediatricians' verbal and phone orders to nurses are not recorded by nurses; pediatricians' verbal orders to the respiratory therapy department are not recorded or communicated to nursing; and/or therapeutic decisions are being made by nonphysicians and are not being recorded.

Organizing Problem Identification Activity

Problem identification activities take place in many different areas of the hospital. The manner in which you coordinate and integrate activities depends on the particular structure of the service, department, or unit and the structure of the hospital-wide quality assurance program.

The organizational framework in which problem identification activities take place will differ from one hospital to another. In every hospital, however, there should be opportunity for at least some departmental review of data as well as some centralized oversight (by an individual, committee, or department). Because the quality assurance standard does not require a specific organizational framework in which problems should be identified, Figure 10 on the opposite page, suggests *only one of many ways* to structure the problem identification process. Regardless of the manner in which problems are identified in your hospital, the organizational structure should be clearly defined. Further, the sites of responsibility for problem identification activities should be specified.

This simplified diagram does not include all services or potential sites for problem identification but suggests a two-way flow between a centralized quality assurance body, which is responsible to the executive committee, and areas in which problem identification can occur. Problems are identified and priorities are set at the departmental, service, or committee level, and information is fed to a centralized quality assurance body. The level of authority of this group can vary from that of a clearinghouse and information center to that of final selection of problems on which the hospital will focus quality assurance resources for a specified period of time.

The methods by which problems are identified in a given service are as varied as the data sources used. However, regardless of the method used to identify problems, it is important to specify both the responsible person at each level and that person's responsibilities for problem identification. In Figure 11 on the opposite page, the data sources used to identify problems related to nursing included information collected from many areas within the hospital.

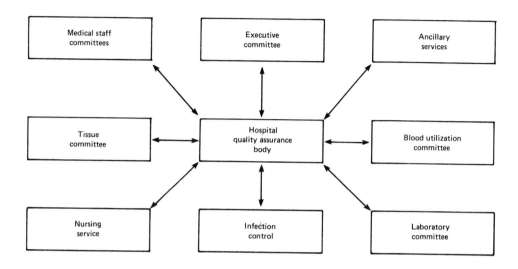

Figure 10. Illustration of one method of organizing the flow of problem identification

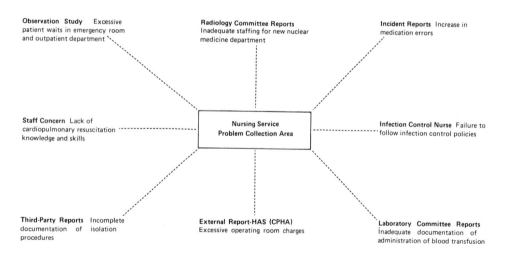

Figure 11. Illustration of the use of multiple data sources for identification of problems related to nursing service.

Exercises in Problem Identification

The exercises provided on the following pages are designed to familiarize you with data sources other than the medical record that have potential use in problem identification. These exercises are designed to assist you to identify

- data sources available in your hospital;
- ten problem areas in your hospital;
- a rationale for the selection of these problems; and
- additional sources that could be used to signal the existence of suspected problems efficiently and economically.

Exercise 1: Identifying Data Sources in Your Hospital

For each of the data sources listed on the opposite page, identify whether it is available in your hospital, whether it is currently used to identify problems, and which quality assurance functions in your hospital use or could use information generated by the data source. For example, morbidity and mortality reports might be available and currently used by the patient care or tissue review committee. On the other hand, staff surveys might be available but might not be used currently, although they could be used by the safety committee, nursing service, and administration, etc. Further, findings of the infection control committee could be used by committees other than infection control.

Exercise 1

Data Source	Available		Currently Used		QA Function
	Yes	**No**	**Yes**	**No**	
Morbidity/mortality					
Tissue review					
Blood utilization review					
Medical record review					
Safety committee findings					
Infection control committee findings					
Prescription review					
Profile analysis					
PSRO regional data					
Incident reports					
Laboratory reports					
Radiology reports					
Financial data					
Liability claims data					
Utilization review					
Staff surveys					
Patient surveys					
Third-party payer data					
Observations					
Other					

Exercise 2: Identifying Problem Areas in Your Hospital

In the space provided, select ten potential problem areas in your hospital and specify the following:
- relevant service or department,
- data sources that could be used to identify the problem, and
- rationale for problem selection.

For example, you might identify an apparent increase in drug reactions on the geriatric service as a potential problem area. Data sources used to identify the problem could include the medical record, pharmacy logs, drug reaction logs, and incident reports. Your rationale for selecting the problem for study might relate to the serious medical and legal complications associated with drug reactions and to the number of services and providers associated with the problem (eg, medical and nursing services and/or the pharmacy department). For an illustration of how two typical problem areas might be described, see page 57.

Problem Areas	**Service/Dept**	**Data Sources**	**Rationale**

Problem Areas	Service/Dept	Data Sources	Rationale
Patient falls	Nursing	Incident reports	Staff on geriatric patient units report an increase in patient falls that result in injury. Because such injuries can extend length of stay and increase the risk of complications (eg, nosocomial infection), the health benefit associated with resolution of this problem warrants review of its extent and probable causes.
Single unit transfusions	Ob/gyn	Committee reports	Reports indicate use of single unit transfusion at a sustained rate of 32-29%, and physicians agree that a much lower rate of use is desirable. The health impact associated with resolution of this concern warrants review.

Figure 12. Illustration of two typical problem areas that might be identified in exercise 2 (see page 56), as well as the responsible service/departments, the data sources used in identifying the problem, and the rationale for selecting the problem study.

Examples of Internal Data Sources

Example 1. *Incident Reports*

Incident reports are an excellent internal source of problem identification data. To use them effectively, it is critical that the information from these reports be organized and displayed so that patterns, trends, and unusual events can be identified easily.

A display of one month's collection of incident reports involving medication errors is shown on page 61.* Twelve incident reports are displayed by patient record number, patient age and sex, physician, nurse, nursing shift, and the number of unmet criteria (based on the criteria illustrated on page 60). Explanations of specific errors are provided under "Notes." To interpret these data, circle the "R"s (requires review), and the following problems become apparent.

- Omission of a medication dose (criterion 6) occurred most frequently (26% of all reported errors).
- Incorrect time of administration (criterion 2), lack of immediate notification of physician (criterion 8), and lack of documentation in the record (criterion 10) occurred with the next greatest frequency.
- Medication errors occurred more frequently in patients of physicians 2 and 3 than in patients of physician 1.
- Errors made by nurses 1 and 5 occurred with more than one patient.
- Errors occurred most frequently on the 11-7 shift, less frequently on the 7-3 shift, and least frequently on the 3-11 shift.
- In 9 of the 12 patient records, at least two errors occurred.

Problems identified in a display such as the one illustrated here, essentially are self-defining. That is, the extent of the problem and the probable cause are determined in the course of problem identification, and no further assessment is needed. Corrective actions can be identified and implemented immediately. Continued collection, display, and monitoring of incident reports constitute reassessment.

The extent to which review of incident reports serves as a simultaneous problem identification and problem assessment process depends on how much information is collected from the incident reports and how thoroughly the information is displayed and analyzed.

(Text continued on page 62.)

---

*Adapted with permission from material developed by Shirley Noah, RN, clinical faculty member, JCAH education programs.

Example 1. *Incident Reports/Medication Errors (Nursing Monitor)*

Purposes To identify patterns in causes of medication errors that indicate prevention measures.

To determine if documentation on incident forms and individual patient records is complete from a medicolegal perspective.

Criteria	Standard
1. If administered, medication administered to right patient	100%
2. If administered, medication administered at right time	100%
3. If administered, medication administered in right dose	100%
4. If administered, medication administered by right route	100%
5. If administered, right drug administered	100%
6. No omission of drug ordered	100%
7. Discontinued or stop-dated drugs discontinued on schedule	100%
8. Physician notified immediately of error	100%
9. Incident reviewed by physician	100%
10. Error noted in patient's medical record	100%
11. Adverse effect	0%
12. Transcription error	0%

Data collected for one month, see table on page 61.

Example 1. *Incident Reports (Nursing Monitor continued)*

Key: X= Meets criterion
R= Requires review
NA= Not administered

Record No.	Age/Sex	Physician No.	Nurse No.	Shift	1	2	3	4	5	6	7	8	9	10	11	12	Notes
																	Criteria
45654	64/M	3	1	11-7 7-3	X	R	X	X	X	X	X	R	X	X	X	X	Gentamycin IV; med card placed in incorrect hour of administration and one dose omitted; team leader (TL) failed to check.
45661	68/F	2	2-4	3-11 11-7	NA	NA	NA	NA	NA	R	X	X	X	R	X	R	Gentamycin 80 mg, q 8 hr; med omitted x two doses by 3-11 shift; 11-7 shift lost med card; Kardex check did not discover error.
45667	83/F	2	3	11-7	X	X	R	X	X	X	X	X	X	R	X	X	Geocillin 250 mg, IV, q 6 hr; ordered wrong dose; administered once.
45772	74/M	3	5	11-7 7-3	NA	NA	NA	NA	NA	R	X	R	X	R	X	X	Tigan 250 mg; omitted 11 am dose; 11-7 shift had in 2 pm slot; TL failed to check.
45776	61/F	3	5	11-7 7-3	NA	NA	NA	NA	NA	R	X	R	X	X	X	X	Phazyme 95 1 tab ac omitted @ 11 am; card in incorrect slot for administration; TL did not check.
45766	61/F	3	5	11-7 7-3	NA	NA	NA	NA	NA	R	X	R	X	X	X	X	Tigan 250 mg qid ac; card in incorrect time slot; not administered @ 11 am; TL did not check.
45917	8/F	2	6	3-11 11-7	X	R	X	X	X	X	X	X	X	X	X	X	Procaine HCL IV given @ incorrect time; med card in wrong slot; TL did not check.
45719	51/F	3	-	7-3	X	X	X	X	R	X	X	X	X	X	X	X	Duplication of med; MD wrote both orders; nursing staff unaware same drug (Ilosone = erythromycin).
45937	4/F	-	7	11-7	X	X	X	R	R	R	X	X	X	X	X	X	Amoxicillin 125 mg po ordered; amoxicillin 125 mg IM given.
45999	28/F	1	13,14	7-3	NA	NA	NA	NA	NA	R	X	X	X	X	X	R	GB series ordered day of admission; Bilopaque not administered; no other preparation.
45970	60/M	1	1	11-7 3-11	NA	NA	NA	NA	NA	R	X	X	X	X	X	X	MD left order for "continue all home meds"; family did not bring meds in until next am; insulin not administered.
46071	8/M	2	5,8,1	all	X	R	X	X	X	X	X	X	X	X	X	R	Transcribed wrong; administered 3 x per day.

Example 2. *Hospital Staff Survey on Areas of Concern for Further Study*

Staff surveys are also an excellent internal source of information for problem identification. Because of staff members' broad knowledge of the day-to-day operation of the hospital, they can help identify important problems or areas of concern for further study.

The staff survey results shown on the opposite page illustrate the broad range of patients, providers, and problems that can be elicited in a survey. After results of this survey were tabulated as shown in the example, the quality assurance committee that conducted the survey determined the frequency with which staff identified similar areas of concern. This step assisted the committee in setting priorities for further study.

Another step that the committee might take before setting priorities or conducting further investigations would be to summarize broad areas of concern. For example, at least three broad categories of concern are evident in the study results: patient education (items 1, 11, 13, 14); criteria development (2, 3, 10, 19, 20); and administrative and direct care issues such as admission and transfer procedures and patient services (4, 10, 17, 18).

Categorization of these areas of concern helps identify problem areas that might affect a larger number of patients than might be obvious when problem areas are considered individually.

Before setting priorities based on staff survey results, it is important to know how pervasive is the concern about specific problem areas. Thus, to avoid lengthy lists of staff "pet peeves," instruct staff involved in a survey to specify areas of concern that have an impact on patient care. A basic definition of impact (eg, serious affect on a large number of patients) should be given.

Example 2. *Hospital Staff Survey on Areas of Concern for Further Study*

1. Patient education required to reduce recidivism rate of chronic obstructive pulmonary disease (COPD)

2. Criteria for use of Holter monitors should be established.

3. Identification of types of effusion and criteria for length of stay (LOS) lacking for pleural effusion

4. Investigate inpatient procedures that could be done on outpatient basis regarding GI admissions

5. Critical patient care events and information flow should be identified

6. Disoriented patients should be investigated

7. High incidence of new decubiti should be studied

8. Diagnosis and treatment of patient with alcohol withdrawal

9. Missed cases of hypertension throughout hospital should be investigated

10. Establish criteria for and study patient perceptions of effort (within hospital) to facilitate patient transfers

11. Investigation of LOS, complications, and education of patients with pacemakers

12. Investigate problems with care of tracheostomy patients, including types of cuffs and complications

13. Study patient education needs and complications of chronic renal failure patients

14. Study problems with diet, education, and complication of diabetic patients

15. Investigate adequacy of medical workup on cases of hypercalcemia

16. Hazards of immobility due to stroke

17. Evaluate emergency room admission process, appropriateness of admissions, and loss of orders

18. Using a "full service" audit, evaluate what services patients might receive that they do not now receive

19. Develop criteria and show justification for use of CAT scanners

20. Develop criteria and useful data on brain scans

21. Investigate appropriateness of use, cost, and efficacy of antibiotics in current use

22. Develop baseline data for myocardial infarction survival study

Example 3. *Patient Survey (Problem Areas for Investigation)*

Like staff surveys, patient surveys are a valuable source of information about problem areas in a hospital. Patient surveys can be conducted by asking patients to complete questionnaires or by conducting interviews in person or by telephone.

The form and content of survey instruments (eg, questionnaires) vary considerably. They might contain open-ended questions (eg, "What problems did you experience while in the hospital?"); rating questions (eg, "On a scale of 1 [low] to 5 [high], where would you place the quality of this hospital's food?"); or forced choice question (eg, "Will you use this hospital again? Yes or no."). Surveys can cover any aspect of hospitalization in as great or as little detail as desired.

In the example of patient survey results shown on the opposite page, Table 1 illustrates the distribution of interviewee's occupations. The professions represented in this survey are fairly evenly distributed, although there is a slightly higher percentage of administrative personnel and a rather low percentage of higher executives and major professionals. Missing from this table is information on how well this distribution reflects the total patient population in the hospital. Although such information might not be critical in a survey to identify problems, the information is necessary if survey results are to be interpreted carefully.

Table 2 illustrates the distribution of the patients' responses to nine questions regarding their experiences in the hospital. Because more than 50% of the responses to items 1 and 4 (satisfaction with preadmission information and with physician) indicate moderate to low satisfaction, these areas should be considered for further investigation. On the other hand, although only 10% of the patients indicated that they would not likely return to the facility again (item 9), it is often useful to explore the reasons for such dissatisfaction.

In items 5 and 6, it is not clear whether patients were to indicate that the amount of discomfort/worry and irritation was high or low or whether their satisfaction with the amount of discomfort/worry and irritation was high or low. Because they are ambiguous and difficult to interpret, these types of questions should be avoided unless specific instructions are given.

Example 3. *Patient Survey (Problem Areas for Investigation)*

Table 1. Distribution of Interviewees' Occupations

Occupational Category	Number	Percentage
Higher executives and major professionals	11	4
Business managers and lesser professionals	31	11
Administrative personnel, small independent businessmen, minor professionals	64	23
Clerical and sales technicians	31	11
Skilled manual employees	37	13
Machine operators and semiskilled	48	17
Unskilled employees	33	12
Never worked or unknown	29	10

Table 2. Indexes of Patients' Ratings of Hospitalization

Index	Distribution of Responses by Percentage				
	High				Low
1. Satisfaction with preadmission information on medical care and costs	3	0	56	36	15
2. Satisfaction with preadmission information on hospital procedure	69	-	8	-	23
3. Satisfaction with hospital food	44	21	-	19	16
4. Satisfaction with physician	56	-	36	-	8
5. Discomfort/worry	24	18	27	20	12
6. Irritation	2	8	-	22	68
7. Satisfaction with information about illness while in hospital	63	17	9	7	5
8. Satisfaction with information about illness after discharge	75	13	-	5	6
9. Likelihood of future use of medical center	83	-	7	-	10

Tables adapted from Houston CS, MD, and Pasanen WE, "Patient Perceptions of Hospital Care," in *Hospitals,* 46(3):71-73, April 16, 1972. Reprinted with permission.

Example 4. *Generic Screening Criteria**

Generic screening or general outcome criteria, if properly used, can provide comprehensive, current, and practical data on patient care and can lead to detection of adverse events that might otherwise be missed. The general outcome screening criteria shown on pages 68-69 cover all aspects of hospitalization and are generally used to screen every patient record. The criteria set was tested during the California Medical Insurance Feasibility Study in 1976 and found effective in identifying nearly all important adverse events that occur in hospitals. Nevertheless, the criteria should not be adopted without consideration of individual institutional needs. For example, some hospitals might add criteria that relate to informed consent or patient dissatisfaction; others might delete criteria that are not particularly applicable to the institution or to a review focused on a specific service or area. Specialty hospitals might add criteria appropriate to their special focus (eg, a psychiatric facility might add criteria to screen for suicide attempts or assault). However criteria are modified, each should serve as a warning flag when an adverse event occurs.

---

*From Craddick JW: The medical management analysis system: A professional liability warning mechanism. *Quality Review Bulletin* 5:2-8, Apr 1979. The criteria originally appeared in the monograph *Medical Management Analysis. A System for Controlling Losses and Evaluating Medical Care.* San Francisco: Marsh & McLennan, 1978. Reprinted with permission.

Example 4. *General Outcome Screening Criteria for Hospitals*

Elements	Standard 0%	Exceptions	Instructions for Data Retrieval
1. Admission for adverse results of outpatient management	X	**1A.** Prior medical care unrelated to this hospital's outpatient department (OPD) or did not involve any member of this hospital staff	**1.** Check admission note. diagnosis. consult notes for complications. failure to treat or prevent or failure to diagnose †
2. Admission for complication or incomplete management of problem on previous hospital admission	X	**2A.** Complication or incomplete management occurred at another hospital **2B.** Readmission for chronic disease, eg. asthma. congestive heart failure, cancer and discharge plan and follow up documented on previous admission	**2.** Check admission note. diagnosis. consult notes; review discharge summaries on prior hospitaliza- tions within 6 months
*3. Hospital-incurred incidents including drug and trans- fusion reactions	X	**3A.** None	**3.** Check progress notes. nurse's notes. consult notes. discharge summary ‡
4. Transfer from general care unit to special care unit	X	**4A.** Scheduled prior to surgery or other special procedure **4B.** Intensive care unit (ICU) used as a recovery room	**4.** Special care = ICU. coronary care unit. respiratory care unit; check orders. nurse's notes. Report reason for transfer and condition on transfer
5. Transfer to another acute care facility	X	**5A.** Mandatory transfer for administrative reasons **5B.** Transfer for test or procedure not available in this hospital	**5.** Report name of facility. reason for transfer. condition on transfer
**6. Operation for perforation, laceration, tear or injury of an organ incurred during an invasive procedure	X	**6A.** None	**6.** Check operative note. progress notes. nurse's notes §

*Report immediately if severe
**Report immediately

† Clues to adverse results of outpatient management include delayed diagnosis (eg. first admission for advanced tuberculosis, metastatic carcinoma; perforated appendix; severe diabetic ketoacidosis; shock; septicemia: any disease with systemic complications); any condition attributed to outpatient drug therapy (eg. digitalis intoxication: hypokalemia while on diuretics; gastrointestinal bleeding while on aspirin. steroids. butazolidine. indocin: bleeding while on anticoagulants; parkinsonism while on tranquilizers; anaphylaxis, drug reactions): complications of procedures performed in the office, clinic or emergency room (eg. malunion, non-union, or complications of fractures; irradiation burns; wound infections; physical defects; neurological defects; complications of physical therapy, x-ray, or laboratory procedures or other outpatient procedures); any disease for which immunization available (eg. measles, mumps, polio, hepatitis, diphtheria, tetanus).
‡ Incidents include medication errors, patient accidents, procedural errors. electrical shock or burn. intravenous errors, drug or contrast material reactions, transfusion reactions, and actual or attempted patient suicide.
§ Invasive procedures include intubations (tracheal, esophageal, gastric. rectal); percutaneous aspirations (thoracentesis, paracentesis, pericardiocentesis, bladder aspirations); percutaneous biopsy of heart. liver. lung. kidneys. prostate, etc; catheterization of bladder, heart, vascular system; x-ray procedures (arteriograms. · renograms, ventriculograms, bronchograms, pneumoencephalograms); endoscopics (bronchoscopy, cystoscopy. sigmoidoscopy, esophagoscopy, mediastinoscopy, peritoneoscopy, laparoscopy, culdoscopy, urethroscopy. ureteroscopy); pacemaker insertion; uterine sounding; enemas; and rectal temperatures.

Example 4. *General Outcome Screening Criteria for Hospitals (continued)*

Elements	Standard 0%	Exceptions	Instructions for Data Retrieval
7. Cancellation of or repeat diagnostic procedure due to improper preparation of patient, technican error or equipment failure	X	7A. None	7. See orders for repeat procedures, nurse's notes, progress notes, lab and x-ray reports, operative notes
8. Unplanned return to the operating room (OR) on this admission	X	8A. None	8. Planned return to the OR must be documented prior to first surgery
**9. Unplanned removal or injury or repair of an organ or part of an organ during an operative procedure	X	9A. None	9. Check operative note, consult form, preoperative plan, and compare with pathology report
**10. Myocardial infarction during or within 48 hrs of a surgical procedure on this admission	X	10A. Preop workup included normal electrocardiogram (ECG) and enzymes and negative cardiac history 10B. Emergency operative procedure	10. Check ECGs, progress notes, consults 10A. Check history, preoperative ECG, lab work 10B. Patient operated on for life-threatening condition
11. Infection not present on admission (nosocomial)	X	11A. None	11. Instructions per infection control coordination; include wound infections
12. Neurologic deficit present at discharge which was not present on admission	X	12A. None	12. Check nurse's notes for seizures, loss of consciousness, impairment of special senses or motor functions, fecal or urinary incontinence, or intractable pain, cerebrovascular accident, stroke
13. Length of stay (LOS) ≥ 90th percentile	X	13A. Increased LOS due solely to nonmedical problems	
**14. Cardiac or respiratory arrest	X	14A. None	14. Assume arrest if code called or any resuscitation performed. Include newborn resuscitation for Apgar ≤ 4 in delivery room
**15. Death	X	15A. None	15. If death occurs, attach mortality review sheet to committee work sheet
16. Other complications	X	16A. None	16. List all not covered by criteria
**17. Subsequent admission for a complication or adverse effect of this hospitalization	X	17A. None	17. Check subsequent admissions history, final diagnosis, consult notes
18. Subsequent visit to emergency room (ER) or OPD for complication or adverse result of this hospitalization	X	18A. None	18. Check ER/OPD visits for unplanned returns for unexpected results

Table 1 originally appeared in the monograph, *Medical Management Analysis, A System for Controlling Losses and Evaluating Medical Care*, published by Marsh & McLennan, Inc, 1978. Reprinted with permission.

Example 5. *Patient Bill*

Patient bills can be used as a data source for problem identification. The patient bill illustrated on the opposite page displays the cost of care for a patient who was hospitalized for 37 days with the diagnoses of cerebro-vascular accident and pulmonary embolism. A review of this bill will indicate the services and level of services that were provided to the patient during hospitalization. Comparison of a sample of bills for patients in the same diagnostic category could determine whether unnecessary or inappropriate services or level of services are a potential problem.

Example 5. *Patient Bill (Diagnosis: Cerebrovascular Accident and Pulmonary Embolism)*

Daily Hospital Service	Amount
4/12-4/14 3 days 332-1 @$ 87.75	$ 263.25
4/15-4/30 16 days 328-2 @ 87.75	1404.00
5/01-5/08 8 days 328-2 @ 94.00	752.00
5/09-5/12 4 days 299 @ 242.00	969.00
5/13-5/16 4 days 298 @ 198.25	793.00
5/17-5/18 2 days 243-1 @ 94.00	188.00
Total daily hospital service	4369.25

By Department	
Cardiac monitor	$ 240.00
Medical/surgical supplies-services	53.25
IV therapy supplies	60.05
Emergency room services	27.70
Immunology	83.40
Lab-urinalysis	33.30
Lab-chemistry	315.50
Lab-bacteriology	178.50
Lab-histopathology	142.80
Lab-hematology	224.70
Lab-blood tests	200.85
Lab-cytology	140.00
Lab-stat	275.80
Blood-bank	265.30
EKG	167.50
Endocrinology	136.15
EEG	90.00
X-ray	498.00
Pharmacy	121.52
Respiratory therapy	44.40
Nuclear medicine	417.35
Ultrasound procedure	65.05
Admission charge	74.45
Patient kit	5.00

Totals	
Total charges	$8229.82
Total adjustments	0.00
Patient payments	0.00
Net balance due	8229.82
Estimated insurance coverage	
Balance due from patient	

Examples of External Data Sources

Example 6. *PSRO/Local Mortality Rates Data*

Data generated by PSROs can be a useful source of problem identification information. The example on the opposite page illustrates data on myocardial infarction and arrythmia rates collected in fifteen 250-bed, acute general hospitals. Rates in each hospital for all patients and for Medicare patients are based on 1977 data. State and PSRO area averages are also provided. Also the number of patients (N) upon which each rate is based is in parentheses.

Data such as these can be used to compare individual hospital performance with similar hospitals in the same PSRO area and statewide. If the individual hospital's mortality rates differ significantly from other hospitals in the area or state, a potential problem exists. In this example, hospitals B and F might consider why their rates are higher for all patients and for Medicare patients; hospitals C and J might consider why their rates are so much lower.

Differences in disease-specific mortality rates do not necessarily mean that problems exist in patient care. Case-mix complexity, socioeconomic status, and patient age should also be considered. Variations in diagnostic coding or in the number of the deaths computed may also account for differences. Once a problem is suspected, an effort should be made to explain the differences during initial assessment. If consideration of case-mix complexity, age, variations in diagnostic coding, etc, yields no acceptable explanation and the problem has been verified, full assessment of the cause of excess mortality should be initiated.

Example 6. *PSRO/Local Mortality Rates*

Myocardial Infarction and Arrythmia Death Rates for 1977

Hospital	All Patients (N)		Medicare (N)	
A	.110	(464)	.136	(198)
B	.215	(65)	.375	(32)
C	.071	(309)	.104	(153)
D	.107	(75)	.108	(37)
E	.107	(467)	.143	(189)
F	.262	(80)	.325	(40)
G	.109	(230)	.154	(130)
H	.124	(250)	.190	(105)
I	.195	(118)	.291	(55)
J	.076	(132)	.125	(56)
K	.174	(459)	.236	(259)
L	.168	(244)	.275	(102)
M	.179	(451)	.299	(214)
N	.173	(567)	.188	(345)
O	.158	(196)	.164	(73)
Area PSRO average	.144	(4081)	.197	(1988)
State average	.150	(9005)	.223	(5698)

Example 7. *Data from the Literature*

Taken from an article on infectious diseases in small hospitals that appeared in the *Annals of Internal Medicine,* the table on the opposite page compares infection rates in 18 small hospitals to infection rates in Hospital X. The table is used here to demonstrate the usefulness of literature as a source of performance standards and comparisons for your hospital. In Hospital X, a larger percent of patient infections were hospital-acquired than were infections in the comparison hospitals. Among the hospital-acquired cases in Hospital X were fewer respiratory tract infections but a greater number of wound infections and infections at "other sites." Based on the assumption that such differences suggest problems, the hospital should explore the problem of wound infection and determine if patterns or areas of concern exist in the higher, "other site" category.

Example 7. *Infection Rates - Hospital Size Comparison* *

	18 Small Hospitals		Hospital X	
	Number	Percentage	Number	Percentage
Total patients	525	100	566	100
Patients with infections	140*	27	107*	19
Community-acquired cases	107		60	
Lower respiratory tract	55	51	18	29
Urinary tract	15	14	13	21
Skin and subcutaneous tissue	13	12	9	15
Wounds	0	0	0	0
Other sites	24	22	22	35
Total sites	107	100	62	100
Hospital-acquired cases	38		48	
Lower respiratory tract	13	33	6	12
Urinary tract	13	33	21	40
Skin and subcutaneous tissue	4	10	2	4
Wounds	5	10	12	23
Other sites	4	10	11	21
Total sites	39	100	52	100

* Some patients had both community-acquired and hospital-acquired infections

*This table was adapted from tables which originally appeared in the articles "Infectious Diseases in Small Hospitals: Prevalence of Infections and Adequacy of Microbiology Services" by Britt MR and "Effects of Infections on Hospital Care" by Dixon RE, printed in *Ann Intern Med* 89(5): 757-760, 749-753, Nov 1978. Reprinted with permission.

Example 8. *PSRO Region, Local, Hospital LOS Profile Data*

The example on the opposite page illustrates a length of stay (LOS) profile for specific diagnostic groups on a regional PSRO, and hospital basis. For each diagnostic category, the LOS in days for the 25th through 75th percentile of patients is indicated by a line. The plus sign (+) at the beginning of the line indicates the 25th percentile; the letter (R, P, or H) indicates the median length of stay; and the plus sign at the end of the line indicates the 75th percentile. The total number of patients upon which the diagnostic LOS profile is based is provided by region, PSRO, and hospital.

Potential problems are signaled when the hospital differs greatly from the PSRO and/or region. The hospital in this example has lengths of stay greater than those of the PSRO and the region in all diagnostic groups, especially in the group "disease of the eye with extraction of lens." Although the hospital's 25th percentile mark begins at or before the median LOS of the PSRO and the region in all other diagnostic categories, the hospital's 25th percentile mark does not occur in this diagnostic category until after the 75th percentile marks of the PSRO and the region.

The hospital should determine why its LOS patterns differ in all diagnostic groups, particularly in the diagnostic group that is so drastically different. The initial part of the assessment of the problem should determine whether unique features in the hospital or variations in management of the data might have influenced the difference in LOS noted between the hospital and the PSRO and region.

Example 8. *Regional, PSRO, and Hospital Length of Stay Profiles for Diagnosis Groups, January-June 1978*

Key:		
	Region	+·····R·····+
	PSRO	+·····P·····+
	Hospital	+·····H·····+

(25th to 75th Percentile; first and last + mark end points; letter marks median

------------------------------- Days Stay · 2 -------------------------------

Selected detailed Diagnosis (DX) group	Total Patients (2)	1 2 3 4 5 6 7 8 9 10 11 12 13 14 15 16 17 18 19 20 21 22 23 24 25
Diabetes, age without (w/o) secondary (2nd) DX		
Region	2063	+·············· R ················+
PSRO	805	+········· P·····················+
Hospital	50	+·················H ·············+
Neuroses, personality disorders		
Region	1387	+···················· R ····························+
PSRO	270	+···················P ····················+
Hospital	27	+···H ·······································+
Eye disease with extraction of lens		
Region	5924	+·······R·····+
PSRO	1405	+·······P·····+
Hospital	110	+·······H·················+
Acute myocardial infarction		
Region	4037	+································R ····························+
PSRO	1187	+···························· P ·······················+
Hospital	50	+·················H····························+
Ischemic heart disease w/o operation (OP) and w/o 2nd DX		
Region	1621	+············ R·······················+
PSRO	730	+············ P·······················+
Hospital	12	+·······························H············+
Cerebrothromboembolism w/o OP and w/o 2nd DX		
Region	1031	+···················· R ·······························+
PSRO	329	+··················· P ·························+
Hospital	11	+···························H································+

Example 9. *PAS Length of Stay (LOS) Study*

The example on the opposite page illustrates the use of the Professional Activity Survey (PAS) data to identify potential problems. In the example, PAS data on LOS are displayed for a specific hospital by physician code (column 1). The total number of the physicians' patients in a specific H-ICDA group is noted in column 2, and the average LOS for these patients is shown in column 3. Column 5 displays the average LOS for similar patients in the same geographic region, and column 6 displays the difference between columns 4 and 5. When the difference is statistically significant, yes is placed in column 7. Column 8 notes how many patients contributing to the difference had *shorter* stays than 95% of the matching patients (under the 5th percentile) and column 9 indicates how many patients stayed longer than 75% of the matching patients (over the 75th percentile). The average stay across the United States for similar patients is noted in the final column.

Ten of the thirty-one physicians were flagged for having patients who remained in the hospital for significantly longer periods than similar patients in other hospitals. The differences in this example range from 3.0 days to 11.6 days. Several of the physicians had only small numbers of patients who contributed to the difference. For example, physician 368 had 14 patients, physician 358 had 15 patients, and physician 324 had 12 patients in this study. Because these data are not adjusted for case-mix complexity and because the size of the samples are so small (except for physician 349), a few patients with unusually complicated medical situations could account for the excess LOS rates. For physician 349, however, at least 49 of his 90 patients contributed to excess LOS, and it is more difficult to find an immediate explanation for this difference in LOS. In all cases, any extenuating factors that might have misconstrued the data should be investigated before further assessment of the causes is initiated.

Example 9. *PAS/Length of Stay Study* *

PAS LENGTH OF STAY STUDY (PHA)

THE PAS BASE DATA

PATIENT GROUP	NO. OF PATIENTS (MILLIONS)
SOUTHERN REGION	3.56
ALL UNITED STATES	14.35
JAN 75 – DEC 75	

. PATIENT GROUP
Reports grouping patients by diagnosis or operation (except summaries) display codes from Hospital Adaptation of ICDA (H-ICDA), 2nd Ed., CPHA, 1973.

. TOTAL PATIENTS
Reports "BY OPERATION" exclude non-operated patients (see list on back of form).

. TOTAL PATIENTS STUDIED
Excludes 1) deaths, 2) patients with age or discharge status not recorded, 3) patients with date of admission or discharge misrecorded, 4) patients transferred to other hospitals, and 5) patients who stayed 100 or more days (although these patients are counted in column 9).

. AVERAGE STAY
The average stay of patients in column 3.

. AVERAGE STAY FOR MATCHING PATIENTS
The average stay of patients similar to those in column 3, taken from the U. S. (or Canadian) regional BASE DATA.

All analyses in columns 5 through 9 use these BASE DATA (see back of form for more detail).

. DIFFERENCE
The difference between the average stays in columns 4 and 5.

. DOES PATTERN DIFFER SIGNIFICANTLY?
"YES" means that the stay pattern for the patient group studied differs, in a statistically significant way, from the pattern for the matching patients. The computer identifies each patient's stay as longer or shorter than the stay for half his matching patients, if the proportion of patients staying longer or shorter is unusually high for the number of patients in the group, "YES" prints. Testing is done at the 5% level of significance.

. SHORT STAY PATIENTS
Number of patients who stayed a shorter time than 95% of the matching patients (under the 5th percentile).

. LONG STAY PATIENTS
Number of patients who stayed longer than 75% of the matching patients (over the 75th percentile). Includes patients staying 100 or more days.

. AVERAGE STAY FOR MATCHING PATIENTS, ALL U.S.
The average stay of patients similar to those in column 3, taken from the all-U.S. BASE DATA.

PHYSICIAN 1	TOTAL PATIENTS 2	TOTAL PATIENTS STUDIED 3	AVERAGE STAY 4	AVERAGE STAY FOR MATCHING PATIENTS 5	DIFFER-ENCE 6	DOES PATTERN DIFFER SIGNIFI-CANTLY 7	SHORT STAY PA-TIENTS 8	LONG STAY PA-TIENTS 9	AVERAGE STAY FOR MATCHING PATIENTS, ALL U.S. 10
296	10	7	14.4	11.2	+ 3.2			2	11.6
297	31	28	18.4	11.2	+ 7.2	YES		15	11.7
303	46	40	17.3	11.2	+ 6.1	YES		24	11.8
306	6	6	11.0	9.8	+ 1.2			3	10.0
308	9	6	18.3	11.9	+ 6.4			3	12.0
309	32	27	14.7	10.6	+ 4.1	YES		10	11.0
310	6	6	20.3	13.6	+ 6.7			5	14.4
314	2	1	5.0	6.8	- 1.8				6.8
324	12	11	13.2	10.2	+ 3.0	YES		5	10.7
326	12	10	9.7	10.5	- 0.8			2	10.8
328	8	8	8.1	9.8	- 1.7			2	10.1
337	8	7	13.1	12.4	+ 0.7			2	12.6
340	2	1	19.0	6.9	+12.1			1	7.1
341	1	1	10.0	16.3	- 6.3				15.4
349	90	73	18.2	11.1	+ 7.1	YES		49	11.4
350	33	31	13.5	9.1	+ 4.4	YES		10	9.6
351	11	10	10.2	9.5	+ 0.7			2	9.8
352	35	33	12.8	11.5	+ 1.3		1	12	11.9
353	43	38	10.1	9.8	+ 0.3		2	11	10.2
356	31	31	12.2	9.5	+ 2.7		1	12	9.9
357	27	22	22.4	10.8	+11.6	YES		14	11.3
358	16	15	15.2	11.5	+ 3.7	YES		6	11.7
359	5	4	9.0	10.1	- 1.1			1	10.1
363	5	5	10.8	8.5	+ 2.3			2	9.0
364	31	30	21.6	10.7	+10.9	YES	1	21	11.0
365	1	1	4.0	6.2	- 2.2				6.4
366	4	2	11.0	8.4	+ 2.6			1	8.7
367	2	2	6.5	8.3	- 1.8				8.8
368	14	14	17.7	11.2	+ 6.5	YES		7	11.7
371	10	10	9.5	7.3	+ 2.2			2	7.3
372	10	7	11.4	9.2	+ 2.2			4	9.8

*This form is reprinted with permission of the Commission on Professional and Hospital Activities, Ann Arbor, Michigan.

Example 10. *PAS Monitor Profile*

An example of a Professional Activity Survey Monitor Profile is illu-
trated on the opposite page. In the first column, the total number of
patients in each group and the percentage of patients who met each
criterion are shown. The second column lists suggested criteria for each
group of patients. Column 3 presents the standard (S) assigned for each
criterion. The profile's columns graphically display the hospital's (H) performance for each criterion, the median (M) performance of other hospitals in the region, and the threshold (T) for investigation (point below
which investigation should occur). An "X" indicates that the hospital's
performance equals the suggested standard. For some criteria, certain data
are "masked" when they fall at the same point on the graphic display (eg,
for the first criterion, "% who died in operating room," the "M" and
"T" are both 0% but are masked by the "X" indicating that the hospital's performance equaled the suggested standard).

In the example, 52% of patients undergoing cholecystectomy in the
sample hospital met the criterion requiring biliary x-ray. The medical
performance of other hospitals in the region was closer to 60% and
further investigation is recommended if the percentage of compliance drops
lower than 90%. In this example, the hospital's performance on two
other criteria (criteria 4 and 5 under "all operated patients") is singled
out for further investigation.

As in any external data sources through which problems are identified, the hospital should decide if factors exist that reasonably account
for the difference in performance. If such factors do not exist, and if
the area of concern is given priority for investigation, further assessment
should be initiated.

Example 10. *PAS/Quality Assurance Monitor Profile**

 EREHWON GENERAL HOSPITAL
ANYTOWN
JUL-SEP
1976

Quality Assurance Monitor
Monitor Profile

Control 5,740,134 PTS, JAN 75 - DEC 75
Group 687 HOSPITALS
U.S. NORTH CENTRAL REGION

PAS
Professional Activity Study

Q Page 1
9798

HOSPITAL PERFORMANCE	CRITERIA — PATIENT GROUPS AND MONITOR PARAMETERS	PATTERN STANDARDS SUGGESTED	HOSPITAL'S	PROFILE
-1-	-2-	-3-	-4-	Hospital Performance H / Hospital Performance Which Meets The Standard X / Suggested Standard S / Threshold For Investigation T / Median (50th percentile) M — 0% 10% 20% 30% 40% 50% 60% 70% 80% 90% 100%
1265 PTS	71. ALL OPERATED PATIENTS			
0	1. % WHO DIED IN OPERATING ROOM	0		X
85	2. % WITH PREOPERATIVE HGB (HCT) RECORDED	100		H ... S
96	3. % WITH PREOPERATIVE URINALYSIS	100		H-S
50	4. % OF PTS OVER 40 WITH CHEST X-RAY (EXCL. OB)*	100		H ... M-----TS
52	5. % OF PTS OVER 40 WITH EKG (EXCL. OB)*	100		H M-------T S
78 PTS	72. TONSILLECTOMY AND ADENOIDECTOMY (CPHA LIST B GROUPS 449-451)			
0	1. MORTALITY RATE (%)	0		X
100	2. % WITH PRO TIME OR OTHER COAGULATION TEST	100		M-X
1	3. % UNDER 2 YEARS OF AGE	0		SH
0	4. % WITH POSTOPERATIVE HEMORRHAGE (998.1)	0		XM
0.00	5. FATALITY INDEX			
LOW	6. WAS PATTERN OF STAY SIGNIFICANTLY DIFFERENT?	NO		
37 PTS	73. PRIMARY APPENDECTOMY (CPHA LIST B GROUP 487)			
0	1. MORTALITY RATE (%)	0		X
17	2. % WITH NORMAL TISSUE*	10-20		S---XS
8	3. % WITH PERITONITIS (540.1)	5-10		SXS M
97	4. % WITH WBC AND DIFFERENTIAL	100		HS
0	5. % WITHOUT PERFORATION WITH PO INFECTION (998.5)*	0-5		XM-S
0.00	6. FATALITY INDEX			
NO	7. WAS PATTERN OF STAY SIGNIFICANTLY DIFFERENT?	NO		
54 PTS	74. CHOLECYSTECTOMY (CPHA LIST B GROUP 497)			
2	1. MORTALITY RATE (%)	0		SH
4	2. % WITH NORMAL TISSUE*	0		S H
94	3. % WITH LIVER FUNCTION TEST	100		M--H--S
4	4. % WITH POSTOPERATIVE WOUND INFECTION (998.5)	0		SMH
52	5. % WITH BILIARY X-RAY	100		H M-------T S
1.88	6. FATALITY INDEX			
NO	7. WAS PATTERN OF STAY SIGNIFICANTLY DIFFERENT?	NO		

*From Lowe JA: PASport. *QRB* 3:20-23, Aug 1977. Reprinted with permission.

Example 11. *Health Services Cost Review Commission Data*

Data generated by a state cost review commission are illustrated on the opposite page. These data display the average charges per case (for the first two quarters of 1978) for patients with disease of the gallbladder and bile duct. Charges are listed for three PSRO areas by type of hospital (ie, rural, urban, and suburban) and by payment category (ie, Medicare, Medicaid, Blue Cross, and others). Total charges for all patients in all payment categories are in the final column in the example. The first number in each column of the five columns is the number of patients on which the average charge was based. The second number is the average charge.

These data are used to compare an individual hospital with similar hospitals in a state. If the individual hospital's charges in each payment category or in total charges differ significantly from other hospitals or from the state average, a potential problem exists. In this example, hospitals B and F in PSRO Area 2 might wish to explore why their rates for Medicare patients (and also for Blue Cross patients in hospital F) differ so much from other urban hospitals in the area. Similarly, hospital L might wish to determine why its rates are uniformly lower.

The initial assessment of a suspected problem should involve a search for possible reasons for the differences, such as whether the hospital included charges for operative procedures and others did not or whether the patient population differed significantly in age, case-mix complexity, or other contributing characteristics from the patient populations in the other hospitals.

Example 11. *Health Services Cost Review Commission/State Charges for Disease of Gallbladder and Bile Duct*

Average Charge Per Case for the First and Second Quarters of 1978

	Medicare		Medicaid		Blue Cross		Others		Total	
	No. of Patients	Charge	No. of Patients	Charge	No. of Patients	Charge	No. of Patients	Charge	No. of Patients	Charge
For Entire Population	891	$3124	268	$2416	1411	$1975	999	$1930	3569	$2282
PSRO Area 1/Rural Hospital	147	$1930	29	$1428	145	$1463	179	$1520	500	$1619
A	37	1466	5	1538	39	1267	32	1109	113	1299
B	3	1103	3	1446	5	2023	4	1443	15	1569
C	13	3230	1	1707	3	1398	14	2200	31	2539
D	18	1548	4	1924	28	1847	29	1830	79	1777
E	32	2443	10	1289	25	1633	36	1954	103	1953
F	44	1775	6	1184	45	1243	64	1198	159	1370
PSRO Area 2/Urban Hospital	265	$4693	120	$3105	453	$2459	197	$2960	1035	$3201
A	0	0	0	0	0	0	0	0	0	0
B	11	9575	15	2510	14	2672	6	2120	46	4195
C	22	3440	13	2115	50	2453	21	2357	106	2597
D	15	3294	2	2079	37	1803	16	1865	70	2145
E	23	6218	14	3355	38	3040	28	4895	103	4297
F	9	9557	9	4628	5	6392	4	3064	27	6366
G	22	3524	9	2927	0	0	0	0	31	3351
H	18	4185	12	5453	49	2435	19	2415	98	3122
I	11	5625	5	2800	20	3570	4	2519	40	3937
J	8	5651	6	3078	15	3497	1	7950	30	4136
K	26	6327	8	3164	55	2483	21	5021	110	3926
L	27	2918	10	2806	57	1991	26	1981	120	2265
M	31	3615	3	2546	65	1821	26	1889	125	2295
N	35	3820	10	1892	36	2716	12	1651	93	2906
O	7	5027	4	2632	12	2531	13	3994	36	3556
PSRO Area 3/Suburban Hospital	70	$3150	15	$2791	101	$1715	122	$2050	303	$2226
A	20	2353	4	2444	32	1454	29	2235	85	1978
B	28	3156	6	2061	53	1847	59	2005	146	2171
C	22	3866	5	3944	16	1801	34	1972	77	2606

Chapter 7. Setting Priorities

When multiple data sources are used for problem identification, as described in Chapter 6, the number of problems that are uncovered can be quite substantial. Because hospitals may have limited staff and financial resources for quality assurance activities and may not be able to solve every problem immediately, priorities should be set for resolution of identified problems. Staff need to develop a systematic approach to problem solving that helps determine which problem areas to explore, in what sequence, and at what rate.

Decisions about which problems to focus on, the number of problems that reasonably can be investigated at any given time, and the order in which they can be investigated and resolved can be made both on a unit/department/service basis and on a hospital-wide basis. To the extent that hospital-wide priorities are set, they should be established by a steering or clearinghouse committee and/or by a group or individual that has authority for oversight of priority-setting activities. Such an organizational structure is useful in that it has the potential to be flexible and thorough, to maximize the effectiveness of resource allocation for quality assurance, to eliminate overlap in problem assessment, and to assure that problems identified at various levels within the hospital are handled in reasonable order. Although the quality assurance standard requires a mechanism for setting priorities, it does not require a listing of problems in order of priority, nor does it require that a specific method for setting priorities be selected.

The main considerations affecting priority setting are the potential impact of the problem on patient care and patient outcomes, and the number of patients affected by the problem. When assigning priorities to problem areas, one should also consider the amount and type of effort needed to complete an assessment. Additional considerations include the impact of the problem on costs, the length of time the problem has been in existence, the number of services or departments involved, staff motivation to solve the problem, and complicated political realities.

Once an estimate of the impact of the problem is determined, the extent of required investigation should be addressed. The effort (ie, time and resources) required to resolve problems varies: Very little time and resources may be expended when problem identification can be followed immediately by corrective action, whereas a great deal of time and resources may be expended when problem identification is necessarily followed by full-scale assessment and monitoring. That is, the process of problem identification is often sufficient in and of itself to allow for the formulation and implementation of corrective actions without additional assessment. An example of this type of assessment would be the routine review of incident reports that highlight an increase in medication errors on a specific nursing unit known to be understaffed. On the other hand, certain problems will be so complex that a full-scale assessment will be required to determine the extent and causes of the problem before appropriate action can be formulated and implemented. An example of such a problem might be a suspected increase in drug reactions. Full-scale assessment might be required to isolate the patient population among whom the reactions are occurring and to isolate the type of drugs, the diagnostic situation, and the indications or contraindications for use of the particular drugs. Between both extremes lie many variations in the effort required to logically assess and resolve a problem.

Setting priorities is an important factor in ensuring the effectiveness and efficiency of a quality assurance program because it facilitates appropriate use of staff time and resources and helps ascertain that problem resolution has a positive impact on patient care and clinical performance. This chapter describes considerations that affect priority setting; outlines methods that can be used to set priorities; and provides an exercise that will help prepare you to set priorities for problem-solving in your hospital (see Exercise 3, page 91). Examples of various methods of, and data sources for, priority setting are provided at the end of this chapter.

Considerations that Affect Priority Setting

Priority setting is a dynamic process. As problems are resolved, new problems will emerge, others will become more urgent, and priorities will change. Therefore, priorities should be revised as necessary, and the ongoing review of multiple data sources and frequent updating of priorities will assist in maintaining an effective quality assurance program that is responsive to identified problems in patient care. In setting your priorities, there are two essential considerations which affect the order in which you should address problems.

- *Impact of the problem on patient care and patient outcomes.*
  The greater the potential for health impacts particularly on

patient outcomes, the greater the need is to resolve a problem quickly.

- *Number of patients affected or potentially affected by the problem.* Again, the greater the number of patients who are or who might be affected by the problem, the greater the importance of solving the problem quickly.

In addition to the impact of a problem and the number of patients affected, there are other considerations that might affect the order in which you address problems. These considerations, outlined below, are applicable only after the previous two priority-setting factors are considered. Problems that involve any combination of the factors listed below should be given a higher priority than those which involve a single factor only.

Duration of a problem. A persistent, serious problem (eg, a steadily increasing nosocomial infection rate) may be given a higher priority than one of recent origin, unless the problem of recent origin is emergent in nature.

Number of services or departments involved. A problem that involves several professional disciplines may be given a higher priority than one which involves fewer disciplines and a smaller number of total providers.

The effort involved in investigating and resolving the problem. A complex problem that requires extensive quality assurance efforts in a setting where resources are limited may be handled in phases. If corrective intervention is not feasible when a problem is identified or assessed, action (resolution) may be deferred until the action realistically can be taken.

Relationship of problems. The extent to which problem areas are related can influence priority setting. A series of problems thought to be related to a single cause may be given a higher priority than a single problem thought to be related to a single cause. For example, medication errors, IV maintenance errors, and faulty preoperative preparation might all be related to poor orientation or inservice education programs in the nursing department.

Staff motivation. Higher priority can be given to problems that exist in areas where staff are well motivated to attain resolution. Success in correcting problems tends to increase motivation among less interested or less motivated staff.

Political environment. The need to respond to problems identified in the accreditation survey process or by regulatory agencies and third-party payers is a reality that should be recognized. Also, the particular interests of influential members of the medical staff and governing body often need to be considered before final priorities are set.

When consideration of the above factors proves insufficient to differentiate priorities, then you should consider the impact of the problem on cost. Problems (eg, excessive use of laboratory tests or single unit transfusion) whose resolution leads to the greatest cost savings without compromising care and outcome should be given high priority.

Methods for Setting Priorities

Setting priorities can be accomplished in various ways. Each hospital must decide for itself what methods of priority setting can be used most effectively at various times and in different areas within the facility. The need for flexibility in selecting and applying these methods is very important. A primary consideration involved in selecting a method for setting priorities entails a decision about the amount of structure or formality required. The priority-setting process can be formal or informal and depends on a number of factors which include the following:

Level at which priority setting takes place. The formality of the priority-setting process is influenced by the level at which priorities are set (eg, unit, department, or hospital-wide), the management style of the responsible individuals, and the number of people involved. Smaller units of service with fewer individuals are likely to find informal methods more practical.

Extent of centralization of the quality assurance program. Because it must organize and incorporate a greater amount of data and because it must be responsive to the concerns of a larger number of people, a highly-centralized hospital-wide quality assurance program will usually require more formal priority-setting procedures than a decentralized program.

Nature of staff relationships and motivation. Well-motivated, reasonably conflict-free staff can deal effectively with informal methods of setting priorities effectively. Formal methods tend to work better when staff turnover is high, when motivation to conduct quality assurance activities is limited, and/or when conflict among practitioners is high.

Approaches to priority setting. The two primary approaches to setting priorities include informal and formal procedures. Informal, non-structured approaches to priority setting include group discussions and committee activity. Unilateral decisions made by one person are probably the quickest method of setting priorities. However, this approach has inherent weaknesses, including a tendency to increase staff resistance and the reduced precision of decisions.

An example of a formal priority-setting method is the structured group judgment exercise or technique. In contrast to group discussion or a committee meeting, structured techniques involve a clearly defined set of operating rules and procedures that specify the framework for discussion, the order and type of participant input, and time limits for such input. These techniques can be used in a face-to-face format or through reiterative written communication. Although written methods

(Delphi techniques) can be used successfully in a health care setting, they are more time-consuming and cumbersome than face-to-face, structured methods.

Informal Priority Setting

If it is to work, the group discussion or committee activity approach to priority setting should be used when the following circumstances exist:

- The task is well-defined. For example, one might say "By the end of the meeting, we will set priorities for these five problems."
- Information available to group members is sufficient to allow them to set reasonable priorities and avoid over-emphasis on personal values (such information should include the extent, duration, and impact of a problem).
- Committee members have knowledge and experience in the areas of concern.
- The group facilitator or committee chairperson is a strong leader who has knowledge of and skill in group dynamics.

Formal Priority Setting

A face-to-face, structured group technique that has been used successfully to set priorities is the structured group judgment technique modified by Williamson* for use in hospital settings. The structured group judgment process eliminates those problems most likely to affect the work of an informal group (ie, lack of task definition, insufficient information, and weak leadership, etc). A structured (formal) group judgment technique is outlined below.

Begin by selecting a group of not less than 5 nor more than 13 people whose combined expertise provides broad experiential input. Lead the group through the following six-step group judgment process; this activity should take no more than 1½ or 2 hours.

1. Allow 5 to 10 minutes for each member to write responses to requests such as "In the time allotted, list problems identified in your hospital (service, unit, etc) and give each problem a priority ranking (weight) 1 through 5." This step provides adequate time for thought, focuses thinking on the question under consideration, and avoids dominance of the group by particularly aggressive, vocal members.
2. Allow 20 to 30 minutes for serial listing of priorities. In sequence, ask each participant to present the most important ideas, one

---

*Williamson JW: Formulating priorities for quality assurance activity: Description of a method and its applications. *JAMA* 239:631-637, Feb 13, 1978. Williamson JW: Priority setting in quality assurance: Reliability of staff judgments in medical institutions. *Med Care* XVI:931-940, Nov 1978.

at each turn, that he or she wrote during the first step, and record these ideas in order on a large flip chart or blackboard. This step allows presentation of all original ideas and stimulates additional ideas. Of primary importance is that everyone have the opportunity to present all of their best ideas.

3. Spend 5 to 10 minutes clarifying the ideas that were listed during step 2. At this point, anyone can ask questions to facilitate understanding of each item. However, do not allow discussion or judgment at this step. Because each person speaks in turn and in order, this step eliminates misunderstandings, highlights the logic behind the ideas, and allows disagreement while discouraging argument.

4. Allow 5 to 10 minutes for each member to record on his or her worksheet a new weight of 1 to 5 for each item listed in step 2 and clarified in step 3. The weight assigned depends on the person's judgment of the extent to which each person meets the following criteria. That is, a) is the problem important? b) is the problem resolvable? c) is having the problem solved worth the effort required to correct it? By eliminating social pressure to agree or disagree, everyone's ideas are preserved. Collect and collate weights from each member for every item and display the results on the flip chart or blackboard.

5. Allow 20 to 40 minutes to discuss the second ranking of ideas obtained in step 4. Judgments and criticisms are allowed in this step of the process. (However, it should be noted that groups generally find that comments which provide factual data are the most useful.) This step assimilates the group's judgments and reduces errors in subsequent interpretations of the group's efforts.

6. Allow 5 minutes for each member of the group to record a final weight for each item. The three criteria listed in step 5 should again be used in making judgments about the final weight assigned each item. This final ranking should be based on the ideas and/or data presented for or against the items discussed. By totaling the sum of assigned weights, the group's final set of priorities can be determined.

Setting priorities can precipitate conflict at any organizational level in the facility. To the extent that individual values can be made explicit, conflict in priority setting can be decreased. The formal method of priority setting that has been described, or a modification of this method, can minimize conflict in establishing priorities. The method not only utilizes a group's total intelligence effectively, but also forces each group member to make his value judgments explicit and stimulates discussion and utilization of facts rather than opinions.

Another method that has been employed in some facilities to set priorites is establishing weights specific to the potential effects of problems. The establishment of these weights forces the group that is setting priorities to make its value judgments explicit and, therefore, is not as useful as a structured group judgment exercise in facilitating conflict resolution. Unlike a structured group judgment exercise, this method relies more heavily on values than hard data. (See page 96 for an illustration of this method.)

Exercise 3: Setting Priorities in Your Facility

Using the problem areas that you identified in Exercise 2 on page 56, and working with colleagues, determine those problems which have the most important impact on patient care and note them in the space below. These would be the problems which you would ordinarily pursue first. Specify the priority-setting method selected and the rationale for selecting those problems which you should pursue first.

Problem Areas   **Priority-setting Method**   **Rationale**

Examples of Setting Priorities

Example 1. *Statewide Data*

The statewide mortality data illustrated on the opposite page are an example of external data generated by a state agency. These data can be used by groups in the hospital to establish priorities for quality assurance topics. Rates are based on 1977 data and have not been adjusted for patient age, case-mix complexity, or socioeconomic status.

The number of patients, the number of deaths, and the death rates in each diagnostic category are provided for the state and for the individual hospital. The asterisks (*) assigned by the state agency indicate diagnostic categories in which the hospital's mortality rate exceeds the state mortality rate by at least 25%, in which at least five hospital deaths occurred, *and* in which the hospital death rate is at least 3%.

The asterisks indicate 12 diagnostic categories that could be considered priorities for investigation: malignant neoplasm of the digestive and respiratory systems; acute myocardial infarction; arrythmia and slowed conduction; heart failure; cerebrovascular diseases; pneumonia; other lung and pleural disease; miscellaneous diseases of the intestine and peritoneum; diseases of the kidney and ureter; symptoms referable to the nervous, respiratory, and circulatory systems; and miscellaneous signs, symptoms, and conditions.

The use of such data in priority setting allows comparison of hospital performance with regional (state) norms and measurement of the amount of difference between mortality rates. However, use of these data is somewhat limited by the arbitrary selection of a 25% standard; the lack of adjustment for age, case-mix complexity, and socioeconomic status; and the difficulty associated with identification of problem sources in broad diagnostic categories such as miscellaneous signs, symptoms, and conditions.

Example 1. *Statewide Mortality Data*

Diagnostic Category	State			Hospital		
	No. of Patients	No. of Deaths	Death Rate No.	No. of Patients	No. of Deaths	Death Rate No.
Infectious disease (dis)	10844	306	3	85	4	5
Malig neoplasm of digestive system	5008	782	16	42	6	24*
Malig neoplasm of respiratory system	3788	731	19	19	7	37*
Malig neoplasm of skin	902	22	2	4	0	0
Malig neoplasm of breast	2742	198	7	14	1	7
Diabetes	6639	119	2	162	4	2
Alcoholic mental disorder & addiction	3966	22	1	46	2	4
Other mental disorders	2253	22	1	11	1	9
Dis of central nervous system	3617	110	3	21	2	10
Dis of peripheral nervous system	3051	1	0	42	0	0
Dis of eye	10032	12	0	35	0	0
Dis of ear & mastoid process	3461	1	0	4	0	0
Hypertensive heart dis	3689	69	2	88	3	3
Acute myocardial infarction (AMI)	7318	1110	15	48	11	23*
Ischemic heart dis except AMI	14849	471	3	177	5	3
Arrythmia & slowed conduction	4497	711	16	32	10	31*
Heart failure	5947	787	13	111	21	19*
Carditis, valvular & other	2511	131	5	16	3	19
Cerebrovascular diseases	8654	1267	15	132	32	24*
Dis of vascular system	9313	478	5	90	2	2
Pulmonary embolism	1286	150	12	22	3	14
Phlebitis & thrombophlebitis	2107	6	0	19	0	0
Hemorrhoids	3131	2	0	33	0	0
Hypertrophy of tonsil & adenoid	12174	2	0	94	0	0
Acute upper respiratory infection & influenza	3078	4	0	13	0	0
Other dis of upper respiratory tract	5402	1	0	19	0	0
Pneumonia	6834	450	7	97	14	14*
Bronchitis	4098	12	0	13	0	0
Asthma	2802	3	0	32	0	0
Other lung & pleural dis	6999	413	6	67	8	12*
Dis of oral cav, salivary glands, jaws	3686	0	0	19	0	0
Gastric & peptic ulcer	3879	57	1	33	1	3
Upper GI dis except gastric, peptic ulcer	4482	21	0	32	0	0
Appendicitis	4303	11	0	25	2	8
Hernia of abdominal cavity	12720	30	0	132	4	3
Entri, diverti, func dis of intestine	4036	34	1	45	1	2
Dis of anus	2832	1	0	33	0	0
Misc dis of intestine & peritoneum	4411	187	4	57	6	11*
Dis of liver	2747	271	10	42	3	7
Dis of gallbladder & bile duct	8453	53	1	68	3	4
Dis of pancreas	1836	33	2	64	1	2
Dis of kidney & ureter	3868	287	7	37	6	16*
Urinary calculus	4366	4	0	18	0	0
Cystitus & other urinary dis	7433	30	0	50	2	4
Normal delivery	25344	1	0	164	0	0
Delivery with complication	19220	3	0	153	0	0
Dis of skin & subcutaneous tissue	6337	42	1	113	1	1
Arthritis	4677	15	0	26	1	4
Derangement of intervertebral disk	5844	4	0	12	0	0
Dis of bone & cartilage	4659	10	0	135	0	0
Other dis of musculo-skeletal system	10249	23	0	454	1	0
Congenital anomalies	4790	57	1	40	0	0
Normal, mature birth	42283	34	0	289	0	0
Certain dis peculiar to newborns	3492	325	9	34	1	3
Symptoms to nerv, resp, & cir systems	8083	169	2	116	5	4*
Symptoms to GI & urinary systems	6493	86	1	31	1	3
Misc signs, symptoms, & conditions	9330	380	4	113	16	14*
Fractures	16974	282	2	191	4	2
Disloc & other musculo-skeletal injury	5371	1	0	9	0	0
Int injury to cranium, chest, & other	4993	221	4	63	2	3
Open wound & superficial injury	7222	55	1	206	3	1
Burn	1136	21	2	15	0	0

*Hospital death rate is at least 25% above state death rate and diagnostic category has at least 5 hospital deaths and a hospital death rate of at least 3%.

Example 2. *Nominal Group Process**

The example on the opposite page illustrates the results of a nominal (structured) group process technique used to identify and set priorities for quality assurance topics with high health impact potential. The topics were selected in an HMO by two independent teams whose members were matched by profession and experience. Structured group judgment was used to maximize the input of experts (ie, individuals deemed knowledgeable about the hospital and its problems) to the problem identification process.

Review of the two lists indicates that the independent teams selected four topics in common, treatment of obesity (A-1 and B-2); identification of sexual dysfunction (A-3 and B-9); care of anemia in infants and young children (A-5 and B-7); and identification of depression (A-10 and B-8). The teams placed three of these topics within two ranks of each other. Team A identified four topics relating to patient education or behavior change and team B selected three topics in those areas.

As evidenced by the range of topics on each list, structured group judgment facilitates representation of diverse groups or interests in a hospital. Furthermore, if one assumes that the process stresses reliance on available facts rather than on feeling, this process also facilitates selection and setting of priorities.

---

*Williamson JW et al: Priority setting in quality assurance: Reliability of staff judgments in medical institutions. *Med Care:* 16:931-940, Nov 1978. Tables appeared on page 939. Reprinted with permission.

Example 2. *Nominal Group Process (Structured Group Judgment Technique)*

Team A Topics

1. Treatment of obesity in patients over 18 in Dr._____'s behavior modification program.

2. Treatment of motivated Type A adult males for Type A behavior by primary care providers and mental health team.

3. Identification of patients with sexual dysfunction by primary care providers.

4. Education for appropriate utilization (of health service) for any patient with any health problem by all providers.

5. Follow-up care of iron deficiency anemia in infants and children by primary care providers.

6. Evaluation of breast mass in women over 25 by primary care providers.

7. Diet change treatment for patients with constipation by primary care providers.

8. Treatment of parenting problems in parents by primary care providers and mental health team.

9. Education of parents for prevention of childhood poisoning in patients under 18 by primary care providers.

10. Identification of depression in patients over 50 by primary care providers and mental health team.

Team B Topics

1. Rehabilitation of enrolled alcoholic teens and adults by primary care providers and mental health team.

2. Behavioral group therapy for weight reduction in enrolled adults over 19 with obesity by mental health team.

3. Dental care provision in plan for enrolled Medicaid patients 4-16 years old with all dental problems by administrators.

4. Education to improve compliance in taking medication in enrolled patients over 30 presently being treated for hypertension by MD and nurse practitioner.

5. Reduction or elimination of smoking by education and therapy in enrolled patients over 12 who are heavy smokers (one or more pack/day) and want to stop or reduce by primary providers and mental health team.

6. Detection of inadequate immunization status in enrolled patients 2 months to 16 years for preventable childhood diseases by MD and nurse practitioner.

7. Etiologic diagnosis of hypochronic microcytic anemia in enrolled and fee-for-service patients 9-18 months by MD and nurse practitioner.

8. Identification of depression in all enrolled and fee-for-service patients by primary providers.

9. Identification and behavioral therapy by sexual dysfunction in enrolled patients over 13 years by primary care providers.

10. Identification of asymptomatic gonorrhea by GC culture with all pelvic examinations of enrolled females 12-40 years by primary care providers.

Example 3. *Weighting*

The example on the opposite page illustrates the use of a weighting system in setting priorities. Table 1 provides disability and social disruption weights that can be used to calculate an overall weight for all patients in a diagnostic category. Table 2 indicates how weights are distributed among more than one diagnosis for a given patient. If, for example, a patient with an acute coronary occlusion has three secondary diagnoses, 40% of the overall weight is assigned to the coronary occlusion and 30%, 20%, and 10% of the overall weight is assigned to the three additional diagnoses in the order of importance of the diagnosis. Table 3 includes the priority rankings assigned to six disease categories based on the weight assignments described in Tables 1 and 2.

Weights can be assigned to any phenomenon or event, and any agreed-upon range of weights can be used. The primary strengths of a weighting system are that the system provides an explicit rationale for setting priorities and makes some of the values underlying priority judgments explicit. The primary weakness of a weighting system is that judgments about relative weights are arbitrary and may not lead to accurate emphasis on areas of concern that have a high impact on care.

Example 3. *Weighting System Based on Patient Discharge Information*

Table 1. Weighting Inpatient Impairment

Disability Weight	
Patient, End-Result	**Weight Assigned**
Hospital days	0.1 (per day)
Complications	1 (per complication)
Death	20
Social Disruption Weight	
Patient Age (yr)	**Weight Assigned**
0 to 9	1
10 to 19	2
20 to 59	3
60 to 69	2
70 and over	1

Table 2. Distribution of Patient's Priority Weight
Among Diagnoses

	Proportion of Priority Weight Assigned to			
No. of Diagnoses	**Dx* 1**	**Dx 2**	**Dx 3**	**Dx 4**
1	100%	—	—	—
2	60%	40%	—	—
3	50%	30%	20%	—
4	40%	30%	20%	10%

*Dx = diagnosis. Diagnoses are in order of importance: Dx 1
is primary, Dx 2 is secondary, etc.

Table 3. Priority Factor Rank for Illustrative Disease Categories*

ICDA Category†	Primary Condition	Overall Priority	Primary Diagnosis	Total Diagnoses	Bed Days in Hospital	Mortality in Hospital	Compli-cations	Social Disruption
42	Acute coronary occlusion	1	6	3	1	1	5	10
66	Pregnancy (uncom-plicated delivery)	2	1	1	2	—	3	1
73	Displaced interverte-bral lumbar disk	5	5	11	3	28	30	6
58	Cholelithiasis-cholecystitis	7	12	18	6	16	17	15
46	Hemorrhoids	9	10	12	7	20	11	8
82	Fractured lower extremity	12	15	34	4	15	22	32

*Computed from 7,599 patient discharges from Rockford Memorial Hospital June and November 1965
†First two digits of *International Classification of Diseases, Adapted* (ICDA)

Reprinted from Williamson JW, Alexander M, Miller GE: Priorities in patient care research
and continuing medical education. *JAMA* 204:93-98, 1968.

Example 4. *PAS Priority for Investigation*

The example illustrated on the opposite page is excerpted from a Professional Activity Study (PAS) Priority for Investigation report. The number in the first column refers to the patient group number: for example, number 74 refers to patients who had cholecystectomy. The second column describes the patient groups and specifies the hospital department that rendered care. In the last column is the total number of patients in the group. According to the number who failed to meet the criteria and the importance of those criteria (eg, mortality criteria are more important than length of stay criteria), patient groups are divided by the need for further study. This excerpt shows only two divisions: "highest priority for investigation" and part of "second priority for investigation." The order of listings within each priority level is not meant to suggest an absolute order for investigation. Whenever further investigation is recommended in the Monitor Profile (eg, for cholecystectomy or for all operated patients), that category of patients is placed in one of the two groups.

In deciding whether to accept the ranking reflected in the example as a basis for setting priorities, consider the appropriateness of the problem areas. Consider them in terms of high health impact and the existence of circumstances in the hospital that might mitigate against the need for further investigation (eg, age of patients, severity of disease, availability of alternate or follow-up care, etc).

Example 4. *PAS/Priority for Investigation*

EREHWON GENERAL HOSPITAL
ANYTOWN

Quality Assurance Monitor
Priority For Investigation

JUL-SEP
1976

HOSPITAL-WIDE

QAM Group Number -1-	QAM Group Name -2-		Total Patients -3-
	HIGHEST PRIORITY FOR INVESTIGATION		
01.	ALL PATIENTS	DEPT PED MED	144
15.	PNEUMONIA, PEDIATRIC	DEPT PED MED	31
07.	PATIENTS GIVEN ANTICOAGULANTS	DEPT MEDICINE	86
09.	PATIENTS TRANSFUSED	DEPT MEDICINE	36
10.	PATIENTS GIVEN DIURETICS	DEPT MEDICINE	163
14.	DIABETES MELLITUS	DEPT MEDICINE	18
25.	ARRHYTHMIA AND SLOWED CONDUCTION	DEPT MEDICINE	17
26.	CONGESTIVE HEART FAILURE	DEPT MEDICINE	27
29.	PULMONARY EMBOLISM (MEDICAL)	DEPT MEDICINE	12
33.	PNEUMONIA	DEPT MEDICINE	35
39.	LAENNEC'S CIRRHOSIS	DEPT MEDICINE	7
01.	ALL PATIENTS	DEPT SURGERY	814
02.	PATIENTS WITH ELEVATED ADMISSION BLOOD PRESSURE	DEPT SURGERY	8
06.	PATIENTS WITH ADMISSION URINE SUGAR POSITIVE	DEPT SURGERY	35
09.	PATIENTS TRANSFUSED	DEPT SURGERY	46
10.	PATIENTS GIVEN DIURETICS	DEPT SURGERY	52
20.	ARTERIAL EMBOLISM (SURGICAL)	DEPT SURGERY	4
34.	FRACTURE OF UPPER END OF FEMUR	DEPT SURGERY	12
36.	CONCUSSION	DEPT SURGERY	13
02.	PATIENTS WITH ELEVATED ADMISSION BLOOD PRESSURE	DEPT OB-GYN	15
06.	PATIENTS WITH ADMISSION URINE SUGAR POSITIVE	DEPT OB-GYN	71
10.	PATIENTS GIVEN DIURETICS	DEPT OB-GYN	10
11.	PATIENTS WITH OTHER DRUG THERAPY	DEPT OB-GYN	8
71.	ALL OPERATED PATIENTS	ALL OPERATED	1265
74.	CHOLECYSTECTOMY	ALL OPERATED	54
75.	ABDOMINAL HYSTERECTOMY	ALL OPERATED	47
77.	CESAREAN SECTION	ALL OPERATED	69
	SECOND PRIORITY FOR INVESTIGATION		
12.	INTESTINAL INFECTIOUS DISEASE, PEDIATRIC	DEPT PED MED	37
14.	ACUTE UPPER RESPIRATORY INFECTION, PEDIATRIC	DEPT PED MED	17
16.	ACUTE BRONCHITIS, PEDIATRIC	DEPT PED MED	13
16.	SCHIZOPHRENIA	DEPT MEDICINE	14
21.	HYPERTENSIVE DISEASE	DEPT MEDICINE	5
22.	ACUTE MYOCARDIAL INFARCTION	DEPT MEDICINE	59
27.	CEREBROVASCULAR DISEASE	DEPT MEDICINE	52
32.	INFLUENZA	DEPT MEDICINE	4
34.	ACUTE BRONCHITIS	DEPT MEDICINE	3
37.	GASTRIC ULCER WITHOUT COMPLICATION	DEPT MEDICINE	3
40.	DISEASE OF PANCREAS (MEDICAL)	DEPT MEDICINE	3

Lowe JA: PASport. *QRB* 3:20-23, 1977. Reprinted with permission.

Chapter 8. Assessing Identified Problems

Assessment of problems is a fluid process that can occur either during problem identification or after problems have been identified. Assessment verifies the existence of a problem and determines the extent and probable causes so that appropriate actions can be planned.

Frequently, the extent, potential impact, and correctable causes of a problem become apparent during the problem identification process, and corrective actions can be selected and implemented without further assessment. For example, if routine review of incident reports on medication errors indicates that doses are omitted with unacceptable frequency on a nursing shift which is severely understaffed, the problem (omission of medication doses), the extent (frequency of omission), and the probable cause (insufficient number of nurses) become apparent during the review process itself. Corrective actions, such as adding staff or reorganizing the medication system, can ordinarily be implemented quickly; and no further assessment is necessary.

However, many identified problems require further assessment to determine the extent and correctable causes. And, because every identified problem is unique in nature, complexity, and characteristics, the methods used to assess such problems will vary. Once priorities have been established (see Chapter 7) for examination of those problems that will require further assessment, you should choose an appropriate assessment strategy (or tailor one or more of the strategies available) to the specific needs of your hospital and the characteristics of the problem to be addressed. In this chapter, we will discuss selecting an assessment method and the factors that influence this selection. Also discussed are selecting an appropriate sample and establishing clinically valid criteria. Clinically valid criteria, which can be established either before an assessment method is selected or in conjunction with the application of a selected method, are discussed at the end of the chapter.

Selecting an Assessment Method

In a generic sense, assessment is the evaluation of written material or of observed performance for the purpose of appraisal. In the past, use of the medical record in a traditional medical audit was the primary mode of evaluation. However, the state of the art of evaluation has evolved to the point where three broad, general categories of assessment can be considered. These include document-based review (eg, review of the medical record, profile data, patient education flow charts, incident reports, financial data, etc); direct observation of clinical performance, of operating systems, and/or of the patient; and dialogue and interviews with patients and/or staff.

Document-Based Review

Document-based review is the evaluation of the process or outcome of care that is reflected in a written document. Documents can be selected on the basis of diagnosis, procedures, mortality, infection, and other parameters of care for which collected, written information is available.

Medical audits, monitoring, incident reports, and utilization review are the most widely used document-based reviews.

Traditional medical audits. Audits are retrospective, criteria-based assessments of the process and outcome of patient care that use clinical records to identify possible problems in the delivery of care. Audits should be performed when the information is likely to be recorded, needs minimal interpretation, and represents care that is generally agreed upon.

Monitoring. A criteria-based review which can be used to ascertain that a specified standard of performance is always met, monitoring is used in many facilities to assess specific elements of care on a routine or selective basis. Monitoring can be performed on a limited basis and discontinued when it appears that the problem which is being monitored no longer exists and is unlikely to recur. For example, the prevalence of single unit transfusions can be monitored on a routine basis or on a limited basis until the problem of excess single unit transfusions has been resolved.

Incident reports. These reports presumably are used on a routine basis in many areas of the hospital to record undesirable events in patient care (eg, medication errors, adverse drug reactions, patient falls, etc). When data from incident reports are displayed in a manner that permits analysis of patterns of incidents and when these data are routinely reviewed, incident reports allow simultaneous identification and assessment of problems. (For an example of how to use incident reports in this manner, see Chapter 6.) Because incident reports reflect care that is current, they tend to be more meaningful to providers than retrospective reviews.

Utilization review. Although sometimes considered a quality assessment method, utilization review is used to identify problems more than it is used to assess problems. Claims forms, clinical records, or clinical record abstracts are examined to determine the appropriateness of admission, length of stay, and the use and amount of ancillary services. Explicit criteria (usually the "average" performance in a local area or geographic region) are used to signal unusual performance. Performance flagged in this manner is reviewed by clinicians (against implicit criteria) for quality implications.

Observation Studies

These studies use human or electronic (videotape, films, etc) recorders to document the actual process of care and to assess compliance with established procedures for care. Observation studies permit a broad assessment of many aspects of care; are unaffected by the problem of data missing from the medical records; and are particularly useful for assessing technical skills (eg, surgical or psychotherapeutic techniques) that cannot be documented in the medical record. The types of observation studies range from those which are systematic and use explicit, preestablished protocols and criteria to those which are based on informal, casual observations.

Interviews

Surveys or interviews are used to obtain information from providers and patients about the process and outcome of care and about any perceived problems in that care. The method uses written questionnaires or preestablished questions during face-to-face interviews and provides an opportunity to obtain important information usually not recorded in the medical record.

Specific assessment methods that have been developed over the years can be considered under one or more of the three assessment categories described above. These methods can be used alone or in combination with each other to assess the extent and correctable causes of problems. Historically, the methods which were developed relied on the use of the medical record, although some incorporated use of observation and interviews as well. Because none of these methods are necessarily problem-focused, they need to be modified by hospitals and expanded to become applicable as problem-focused methods. (For an explanation of several of these methods, see Appendix C.)

Some of these methods are more appropriate than others for assessment of particular problems. Some assessment strategies are simple, straightforward, practical, inexpensive, and fast, although they tend to be less sensitive than the more complex, time-consuming, and expensive strategies. An excellent rule of thumb is to select the simplest, fastest, and least expensive method that will yield all the information you will need to plan and implement reasonable corrective actions.

Factors Influencing Selection of Assessment Methods

Because the effectiveness and efficiency of the assessment method are important, the following factors should be considered when selecting a specific method.

Number of issues involved. Multiple, related problems may require greater effort and more complex assessment than single problem areas. For situations in which numerous issues are involved, assessment methods that analyze patterns of care may be more applicable.

Number of disciplines involved. The greater the number of disciplines involved, the greater the effort and the more complex the assessment required. For situations in which numerous disciplines are involved, multidisciplinary or independent studies which evaluate care related to all involved disciplines are more applicable than those which rely on tracking the practitioner's individual logic and clinical decision-making.

Probable extent of the problem. A persistent, widespread problem that has a high impact on patient care may require a large, complex assessment effort to isolate correctable causes and identify corrective actions. A number of assessment methods such as selected observations and interviews can be used simultaneously to determine the extent and correctable causes of a problem.

Type of problem. Certain problems, such as those involving techniques of care or interpersonal relationships (eg, proper intravenous maintenance, performance of cardiopulmonary resuscitation, or preoperative patient education), might necessitate observation studies rather than record-based review.

Audience for results. Quality assurance requirements differ in amount, format, and precision of assessment data and results. Thus, certain external agencies might require that a significant amount of specified data be collected over a particular time period. The hospital, on the other hand, might require only enough data to allow approximate estimates of the extent and probable cause of the problem.

Characteristics of data. Regardless of the data source, certain characteristics of data influence the type of assessment method chosen, the ease with which a study can be conducted, and the effectiveness of a study. These characteristics include availability, accessibility, and quality. The medical record, for example, is a readily available and accessible data source, but such data often are of poor quality (eg, incomplete, illegible). On the other hand, although data on techniques of care (eg, surgical techniques or psychotherapy) can be complete and of high quality when obtained through rigorous observation studies, they are less available and accessible. Thus, assessments based on these data are more difficult to accomplish than those based on medical records. Similarly, high quality data that are valid (ie, measure what they purport to measure) and reliable (ie, consistent) are less complex to interpret and analyze because adjustments do not have to be made to correct deficiencies in the quality of data.

Selecting an Appropriate Sample for Study

Ordinarily, the assessment method you select determines the data source that will be used in the study. In traditional, retrospective medical audits, for example, information is collected from patient records to determine whether the record documents care that complies with preestablished criteria. Medical records always serve as the data source for these reviews. Patient or practitioner comments on problems in medical care are data for assessment that are gathered through a questionnaire or survey. Routine pharmacy reports are a source of information on the types of pharmaceuticals used and the frequency with which they are prescribed.

Census versus Sample

When the data sources for a study have been selected and the assessment method determined, you must decide how many cases (eg, records, questionnaires, or patients) have to be examined to obtain reasonable conclusions. Is it necessary to review all cases or will review of a sample of cases suffice?

A study or assessment that encompasses the entire population (ie, all cases that are potentially relevant to a particular study) is a census. Theoretically, a census provides the most complete picture of the quality of medical care in the clinical setting, because every patient affected (eg, all patients with myocardial infarction) and every practitioner participating in the care of these patients (eg, all cardiologists) are included in the review. A census, however, is not always feasible or desirable. The expense of retrieving every record and the time required to abstract and evaluate the data is often prohibitive. In addition, because so many records might be excluded from the study because they are incomplete, illegible, or have other complicating factors, those which are finally included can constitute a biased sample and cause the assessment to be biased also. Fortunately, many sampling techniques have been developed that allow you to draw the same conclusions from your study results as you would from a census.

The purpose of sampling is to permit you to arrive at valid conclusions about an entire population from data collected solely from a representative sample of the population. The process of drawing conclusions about a population from an assessment of a representative sample of that population is called inference. If sampling techniques are not carefully and accurately employed and/or if the sample is different in some characteristic from the whole population, then the inference drawn from the sample data will be incorrect. Consequently, to make valid inferences from the sample about the population, it is important that the sample be clinically representative of the population. That is, the cases examined must have the same characteristics as the population of interest, and they must have received their medical care in the same location during the same period of time. For the most part, in these types of assessment activities, it is necessary only to be aware of possible biases and make an effort to avoid them.

The decision of whether to use a sample or a census, however, must be made in the context of the particular clinical problem to be examined. If you decide it would be appropriate to use a sample, you must then decide how many cases you will have to study to obtain valid conclusions. Statistical and clinical concerns must be considered when you make this decision.

Significance of clinical concerns. Clinical considerations are involved in decisions about sample size. Certain situations require assessment of a large number, indeed sometimes all, of the possible cases. For example, if a problem occurs infrequently but could precipitate, or is associated with, a grave medical outcome, you will most likely want to conduct a census. Such problems might include emergency medical conditions or other life-threatening situations that might be the focus of medicolegal investigations. These problems are usually so rare that sampling procedures might miss the one or two cases that are most important to elucidating pertinent events and to revealing probable problem causes. Thus, in grave clinical situations, it might be appropriate to conduct a census in the immediate location and immediate time period of the suspected problem.

Even when the situation is less than life threatening, the financial or legal implications of a suspected problem may be so important to an institution that many, if not all, cases would need to be assessed. Further, when it is highly probable that more data will be sought during the course of the study to determine the possible causes of a problem, a large sample, or the total population, might be assessed. Although a few characteristics of the problem may lead to selection of large samples, there are statistical processes that, in most situations, help minimize the necessary sample size.

Significance of statistical concerns. Statistics are utilized to assure that the data sources in the sample (eg, records, patient questionnaires) represent the population under study and that inferences drawn from the sample contain an acceptably low level of error. (Some error is always possible when drawing conclusions about a whole population from a sample.)

Many assessment methods focus on the percentage or proportion of a sample that fails to meet a criterion. For other assessment methods, it is the frequency of undesirable incidents in the sample that is of prime concern. Using the data available from the sample, the percentage or the frequency of these events is calculated. This percentage or frequency is then used as an estimate of the percentage or frequency within the population, with the proviso that this estimate is actually plus or minus a small "sampling error." Using probability sampling procedures, a minimum sample size can be determined without any knowledge of how uniform the patient characteristics are throughout the population under study. When reliable sampling procedures are used, 20 to 30 cases are thought to be the lowest possible sample size that is useful; however the larger the sample, the smaller the error or bias the sample is likely to have.

Probability Sampling Techniques

Use of probability sampling techniques assures that each case in the population has an equal and independent chance of being selected so that, if large enough, the sample has a definable probability of being representative of the entire population. Therefore, from these samples, inferences can be made about the population of primary concern to the investigators.

The following factors should be considered in selecting the sample:
- the characteristics of the population that the sample must represent;
- the location and time of concern from which the sample must be drawn; and
- the type of sampling technique that will assure that the sample accurately represents the population.

To ascertain that the sample contains representative cases, the following procedures can be employed in selecting the sample. All probability sampling procedures begin with a list of every individual in the population from which you will select the sample.

Simple random sampling. In simple random sampling, you select a predetermined number of cases from a list of every case in the defined population (eg, 10% of all patients admitted to the hospital in one year).

Stratified sampling. Stratified sampling refers to dividing a defined population into homogeneous groups or strata according to such characteristics as service, diagnosis, unit, and payment category, and then selecting a sample of predetermined size from each stratum. For example, if one were assessing nursing care of patients on IV therapy, one might sample and assess cases from each nursing unit, nursing shift, and diagnosis.

Systematic sampling. Systematic sampling refers to random selection of only one case. Then a fixed interval is determined and every case at the selected interval after the first case is selected for the sample (eg, every 20th emergency room admission after random selection of the first case). This method is easier than numbering every case and selecting each on a random basis.

Nonprobability Sampling Techniques

Earlier, we discussed how clinical considerations might increase the sample size when the problems being studied were grave but rare. We must now discuss the application of clinical judgment to situations in which the problem is suspected to be quite common; that is, situations in which the prevalence of the problem is thought to be large. The prevalence of a problem is the number of cases reflecting the problem at any given time.

When the problem is quite common, such as arrhythmias among myocardial infarction patients, it is possible to use clinical judgment to reduce the sample size requirements. This is done on the assumption that the situation is so common that an examination of even a relatively few cases will reveal the prevalence of the problem and its probable sources. It is also assumed that the problem is uniform wherever it occurs and that the cases are uniform in most relevant characteristics.

In these instances, nonprobability sampling techniques can be used. These techniques permit the selection of a sample that is somewhat typical, if not absolutely representative, of a known population. However, caution must be used in making inferences from this type of sample to the total population. These sampling techniques include the following.

Chunk sampling. Chunk sampling refers to selection of convenient sections of a population (eg, all patients discharged from a given unit in a particular time period, such as one week).

Purposive sampling. Purposive sampling refers to selecting cases for specific purposes and for measurement against specific, predetermined criteria (eg, all patients over 70 years admitted for corneal transplants in the past year).

Quota sampling. Quota sampling refers to selecting specified numbers of cases from defined classes (eg, 20% of 50 male patients over 65 years of age with a discharge diagnosis of congestive heart failure, or 5% of 25 male patients over 65 years of age with a discharge diagnosis of acute myocardial infarction).

In the interest of efficiency, most review committees will select the smallest useful samples. However, in no cases should the number of cases be less than 20 or less than 5% of the expected population, whichever is greater.

Establishing Clinically Valid Criteria

Clinically valid criteria, which can be established either before an assessment method is selected or in conjunction with the application of a selected method, are statements about the structure, process, or outcome of care drawn from the best in knowledge and experience of experts and from the health care literature. As statements of expected elements of care or expected patient outcome, they are compared with actual practice and outcome. Clinically valid criteria should be established in a rigorous manner, and should be developed and agreed upon before an assessment is conducted. Such criteria should be objective and explicit (ie, written and made available to those whose activities are being assessed). Implicit criteria are based on personal judgment and are not necessarily documented or subjected to review by peers. Although such criteria may on occasion be valid, personal judgment, lack of documentation, and lack of review by peers might introduce subjectivity and compromise assessment results.

The establishment of objective, clinically valid criteria is based upon the professional experience and judgment of acknowledged experts and the relevant, current literature. The standards of practice of professional organizations can be useful guides in the absence of other literature. Involved clinical staff should be familiar with and understand the criteria.

In addition to being valid, criteria must also be specific and measurable. Much assessment time and effort can be wasted if criteria lack necessary specificity. If the specificity or validity of a criterion is in question, the criterion can be tested in a "mini" sample before it is used in an extensive assessment. Pretesting a criterion can be accomplished by selecting a fraction of the sample that might fall into the final assessment and checking that fraction against the criterion for the following characteristics.

- *Accessibility.* The data which is sought should be readily available and easily abstracted. If it is difficult to find the necessary data, the wording and intent of the criterion might not be specific enough.
- *Applicability.* The data which is sought should be present in the record. For example, a criterion concerning patient education might be valid. However, when patient education takes place but is not documented in the record, the criterion cannot be used in a record-based review because the required information is not present.
- *Validity.* Validity indicates the extent to which a criterion measures authenticity. That is, if a criterion calls for an expected behavior or outcome that is not recorded in any of the records, it is possible that the criterion is not valid. The criterion should be returned to the committee for additional consideration. If the committee determines that the criterion *is* valid and that the requisite behavior is not occurring, a problem exists. This reconsideration of the criterion minimizes the possibility that a full assessment will be conducted with an invalid criterion.

Comment

The assessment method you select, the sample you choose, and the criteria you establish will depend on the characteristics of the problem and the resources available for assessing it. The Joint Commission on

Accreditation of Hospitals does not endorse any particular method or methods for assessing problems. The quality assurance standard emphasizes flexibility and is designed to encourage application of a wide range of assessment strategies which are selected and implemented based on individual hospital needs, resources, and/or the type and probable extent of problems under consideration.

The Use of Incident Reports and Observation Studies in Assessing Identified Problems

Example 1. *Incident Reports: Nursing Study of Patient Falls**

Tables 1-6 on pages 111-113 demonstrate the use of incident reports in identifying and assessing the probable cause of 53 patients' falls which occurred in one hospital during a one-year period. Using additional data from the medical record on patient medications, on diagnoses (primary and secondary), on mental status, and on number of days from time of admission that falls occurred, the hospital that conducted this study was able to reach conclusions about patients at higher risk of falls. Based on these conclusions, the hospital was able to take actions to prevent and correct further risk of falls to this patient population.

---

*Walshe A, Rosen H: The study of patient falls from bed. *JONA* 9:5, 31-35, May 1979. Reprinted with permission.

Example 1. *Incident Reports*

Table 1. Patient Falls From Bed by Age and Shift

Age	Shift					
	7-3		3-11		11-7	
	Number	Percent	Number	Percent	Number	Percent
Under 60	1	14.3	3	42.9	3	42.9
60-65	0	0.0	0	0.0	2	100.0
66-75	4	20.0	5	25.0	11	55.0
76-84	1	7.1	11	78.6	2	14.3
85+	3	30.0	4	40.0	3	30.0
Total	9	17.0*	23	43.4*	21	36.6*

*Percentage of total falls per shift

Table 2. Medications Within 24 Hours Before Fall From Bed

Medication	Number of Patients	Percent of Total Patients
Diuretic	27	43.4
Cardiac	19	35.0
Sedative	17	32.0
Antibiotic	11	18.8
Analgesic (narcotic)	7	13.2
Anticonvulsant	6	11.0
Hypertensive	4	7.5
Diabetic	2	3.7

Example 1 (continued).   *Incident Reports*

Table 3. Breakdown by Diagnosis of Falls From Bed

Diagnosis	Primary Diagnosis		Secondary Diagnosis	
	Number of Falls	Percent	Number of Falls	Percent
Cardiovascular	21	39.6	12	22.6
Cancer	7	13.2	3	5.7
Orthopedic	8	15.1	3	5.7
General medical	7	13.2	8	15.1
Neurological	10	18.9	3	5.7
Total	53	100.0	29	54.7

Table 4. Breakdown of Falls From Bed by Age and Side Rail Status

Age	Side Rail Status					
	Up		Down		Unclear	
	Number	Percent	Number	Percent	Number	Percent
Under 60	4	57.1	3	42.9	0	0.0
60-65	2	100.0	0	0.0	0	0.0
66-75	7	35.0	8	40.0	5	25.0
76-84	5	35.7	3	21.4	6	42.9
85+	9	90.0	0	0.0	1	10.0
Total	27		14		12	

Example 1 (continued). *Incident Reports*

Table 5. Patient Falls From Bed by Age and Mental Status

Age	Mental Status					
	Normal		Disoriented		Agitated	
	Number	Percent	Number	Percent	Number	Percent
Under 60	4	57.1	2	28.0	1	14.3
60-65	0	0.0	0	0.0	2	100.0
66-75	11	55.0	9	45.0	0	0.0
76-84	8	57.1	6	42.9	0	0.0
85+	3	30.0	7	70.0	0	0.0
Total	26		24		3	

Table 6. Falls From Bed by Number of Days Since Admission

Day of Fall	Number of Falls	Percent of Total Falls
Day of admission	3	5.7
Day 2	4	7.5
Day 3	6	7.5
Day 4	3	5.7
Total within first 4 days	16	30.2
Days 5 through 11	11	20.7
Total within first 11 days	27	50.9
Days 12 through 100	26	49.1
Total	53	100.0

Example 2. *Observation Study**

Certain aspects of patient care and clinical performance are amenable to assessment by direct observation only. Direct observation allows evaluation of actual performance and measurement of how well a practice, behavior, or procedure was performed, rather than whether it was performed or not. Interpersonal interactions during patient edcuation, specific techniques (such as IV maintenance therapy), and certain systems problems (such as traffic patterns in the operating room) are best assessed by observation.

The observation study illustrated on pages 115-117 was conducted to evaluate the performance of hospital personnel during cardiopulmonary resuscitation (CPR), and to determine whether the hospital meets current standards of the American Heart Association for performance of CPR.

To assure that the study was as objective as possible, questions were designed to require yes or no answers whenever possible. When judgment was required, such as in item A which concerns techniques, precise definitions were provided. Note that observation studies should be conducted by trained personnel who are knowledgeable in the area under observation. (For an example of an observation study using an algorithm or criteria map, see Appendix C.)

---

*Stanford University Hospital Department of Nursing Observation Study, Topic Area—Cardiopulmonary Resuscitation. Reprinted with permission.

Example 2.   *Code 66 Evaluation Form*

A. AHA Standards for Performance of cardiopulmonary resuscitation (CPR)

	Yes	No

1. Were proper techniques of CPR observed?

    a. Body position*

    b. Hand position*

    c. Depth of compression*

    d. Rate of compression*

    e. Compression to ventilation ratio*

    f. Respirations sufficient for chest to rise

    g. Chest auscultated after intubation

    h. Patient's back on firm surface

    i. Respiration and pulse checked every minute

    j. CPR interrupted for more than 5 seconds?
       If so, how long ?_____

> **Exceptions:**   15 seconds allowed for 1) intubation, 2) moving patient up or down stairway or transferring to stretcher, 3) central line insertion

B. Efficiency of Performance of Personnel

1. How soon did the following personnel arrive (within 3-5 minutes)? Did they announce their arrival ?

    a. Pharmacy   _____ min.

    b. Unit manager   _____ min.

    c. Nursing supervisor _____ min.

    d. Medicine   _____ min.

    e. Anesthesiology   _____ min.

    f. Respiratory therapist _____ min.

    g. EKG technician   _____ min.

2. Did one physician assume "charge" of the code?

3. Did one RN assume "charge" of nursing personnel?

    a. One nurse remained with patient and physician

    b. A nurse recorder or pharmacist reminded physician in charge of time sodium bicarbonate, epenephrine, etc, had been given

    c. One "runner" for supplies

4. How many people responded?_____

*See page 117 for explanation of techniques of CPR

Example 2. *Code 66 Evaluation Form (continued)*

	Yes	No

5. If excessive numbers of people responded, were nonessential persons asked to "clear the area"?

6. Other patient(s) in room attended to?

   a. Curtains pulled

   b. Moved out

   If "no," explain_____

7. Equipment and supplies

   a. Space available for optimum performance in caring for the patient?

   b. Modules placed in optimum locations for use?

   1. Respiratory module placed at head of bed
   2. IV module placed at foot of bed
   3. Drug module (crash cart shelf) not placed on bed

   c. All supplies needed during code on crash cart?
   1. How many trips out of room?_____
   2. Specific items sent for included_____

   d. Supplies missing from the crash cart?
   If "yes," what?_____

   e. All equipment functioned properly?
   If "no," explain_____

8. Use of defibrillator

   a. Paddles properly prepared (ie, application of Redux or use of saline soaked pads)?

   b. Operator assured that all persons were clear of patient, bed, etc, before discharging paddles?

9. Family considerations

   a. If family *not* present at time of arrest, notified patient condition worsened?

   b. If family present at time of arrest, escorted from room and kept informed during the code?

10. Patient status after CPR (circle one)

   a. Responsive

   b. Nonresponsive

   c. Expired

11. Additional comments

Signature of observer _____

Example 2. *Code 66 Evaluation Form (continued)*

To be completed by medical records auditor

Patient status at time of discharge from hospital (circle those that are applicable)

1. Alive

2. Ambulatory

3. Nonambulatory (explain)_____

_____

4. Expired

Explanation of CPR Techniques

A. Body position

Rescuer's shoulders directly over victim's sternum.

Elbows straight.

Pressure applied vertically downward on lower sternum, using upper part of body for weight and leverage.

B. Hand position

1. Adults

Place long axis of heel of one hand parallel to and over long axis of lower one-half of sternum. Then place other hand on top of first, 1 to 1½ inches away from tip of xyphoid process.

Fingers should not rest on victim's ribs. Interlocking fingers of both hands will help avoid this problem.

Heel of hand should not be removed from chest during relaxation between compressions.

2. Young children

Heel of one hand only over midsternum.

3. Infants

Tips of index and middle fingers used over midsternum.

C. Depth of compression

1. Adults: 1½ to 2 inches.

2. Young children: ¾ to 1½ inches.

3. Infants: ½ to ¾ inches.

D. Rate of compression (Compressions must be regular, smooth, and uninterrupted.)

1. Adult: Overall, 60 compressions per minute.

2. Young children: 80 to 100 compressions per minute.

3. Infants: 100 to 120 compressions per minute.

E. Compression to ventilation ratio

1. Adults: one-man rescue, 15:2; two-man rescue, 5:1.

2. Small children and infants: one man rescue, 5:1.

Chapter 9. Determining Problem Causes and Corrective Actions

Several recent studies* have shown that two of the most common corrective actions in quality assurance activities are sending a letter citing deficiencies to the medical staff and conducting continuing education programs. These studies also indicate that such actions typically are ineffective.

Before corrective action can be specified for a particular problem, the following three aspects of the problem must be identified:

- site (eg, service, unit, or patient group),
- audience (responsible party or parties)—eg, an individual nurse or physician or a particular group of clinicians, and
- nature (eg, knowledge gap).

Although quality assessment activities usually result in identification of the site and audience, further investigation is often required to determine the nature of the problem. There are three basic categories of problem determinants (causes) that define the nature of a problem.

- *Knowledge.* This category covers problems of a technical or procedural nature. Examples of technical problems would be improper maintenance of IV therapy or unknown synergistic effects of specific drug combinations. Instances of procedural problems would include the manner in which a patient transfer is completed or in which incident reports are reported and recorded.
- *Performance.* Even if practitioners have the appropriate knowledge, the desired performance may not occur because habits, attitudes, or intrapersonal and interpersonal stress exist among staff. For example, practitioners may have knowledge of drug

---

*Kaplan, KO: Analysis of follow-up component of MCE study cycle. HCFA contract 24-77-0074. Kappa Systems, 1977.

interaction but may not apply this knowledge effectively in patient care.

- *Systems.* Even if the desired knowledge, habits, and attitudes are present, problems that prevent appropriate performance may arise from organizational, administrative, or environmental factors. Examples of these factors would be a poorly managed laboratory or pharmacy; a lack of, or inappropriate, staffing; and a lack of, or dysfunctional, equipment.

To be effective, strategies for correcting problems in patient care and clinical performance should be based on accurate assessment of the nature of the problem. Inservice education, for example, will not improve documentation practices if a poor medical record system inhibits those practices. Similarly, a continuing education program on utilization of laboratory tests will not decrease excess utilization if practitioners habitually order an SMA-24.

Corrective Actions

A problem that falls into more than one of the knowledge, performance, and systems categories described above might necessitate a variety of corrective actions. For example, inappropriate usage of antimicrobial agents might reflect any or all of the following:

- lack of provider's knowledge of indications for drug usage;
- long established habit (performance), for example, prescribing a sulfa drug for urinary tract infections without culture or sensitivity (C&S) or before review of C&S results; and
- inefficient laboratory system, for example, C&S not reported in a timely manner.

Although a problem can have many causes, not all causes are amenable to correction; and most problems, to be corrected, require varying amounts of effort. Carefully defining the site, audience, and nature of a problem allows you to focus on problem determinants (causes) that can actually be changed within the available resources, and whose change will result in the most benefit to patients. For example, a million dollar addition to the emergency room (ER) might have to be delayed for financial reasons, but an effective triage system can be initiated immediately to reduce unnecessary ER mortality.

Once the site and nature of the problem and the audience for corrective action have been established, appropriate individuals should develop plans for action that

- describe all actions to be taken;
- assign measurable objectives for each action, including the expected change, the person, group, or situation expected to change, how much change is expected, and the time frame in

which change is expected to occur;
- delineate the person(s) responsible for implementing action; and
- specify when reassessment should take place.

Strategies to Correct Problems

Strategies to correct problems in patient care and clinical performance can be classified in several ways. The following three generic types of strategies* provide a useful framework within which strategies for change can be selected. Although the terminology used to describe these strategies might be unfamiliar, do not be intimidated. The components of these strategies are certainly familiar to you.

Rational-empirical. These strategies are based on the assumption that people are rational, motivated by self-interest, and willing to change if it can be demonstrated logically that they will benefit from change. Strategies in this category include, but are not limited to,
- education (inservice or CME),
- operations research and systems analysis (management tools using quasimathematical models to describe organizational structure and function and to provide more effective, efficient models), and
- other research and development activities (applied research designed to provide solutions to "real world," day-to-day problems).

Normative-re-educative. These strategies are based not only on the assumption that people are rational but also that behavior is supported by the value systems and sociocultural norms of peer groups. Change will occur based on the extent that attitudes, values, goals, skills, and relationships change along with the base of knowledge affected by rational-empirical strategies. The strategies in this category include, but are not limited to,
- language clarification,
- sensitivity training,
- counseling,
- conflict labs (training and simulated experience in dealing with conflict), and
- organizational changes that support alterations in values, attitudes, etc.

Power-coercive. These strategies are based on use of power—which is sometimes legitimate and not legitimate at other times—to effect compliance. Strategies in this category include, but are not limited to,

---

*Chin R, Benne KD: General strategies for effecting change in human systems. In Zaltman G, Kotler P, Kaufman I, (eds): *Creating Social Change.* New York: Holt, Rinehart, Winston, 1972.

- negotiations,
- administrative rulings,
- judicial decisions that change laws, and
- alterations in the power structure.

Ideally, the change strategies you select will be based on the type and nature of the problem identified and the resources available to bring about change. Rational-empirical strategies, such as inservice and continuing education programs, work best when the problem is one of knowledge. Rational-empirical strategies such as operations research and systems analysis work best when the identified problem involves systems and organizational structure. Performance problems are most amenable to normative-re-educative strategies such as sensitivity training and counseling. Power-coercive strategies are most effective when the identified problem involves organizational and management structures, but generally are used only when all other strategies have failed.

These strategies often are used in combination to bring about change. For example, a combination of inservice education (rational-empirical) and sensitivity training (normative-re-educative) for nurses may be the most powerful change mechanism for a problem in the education and counseling of terminally-ill patients.

Guidelines for Motivating Change

Once you have selected an overall strategy for corrective action and change, consider using the hints described below to maximize the potential for achieving change. These hints are based on guidelines for motivation developed by several psychologists interested in social change, including Doob.*

Involve staff early, if only by informing them of assessment efforts and progress. People are interested in their own discoveries and respond better to their discoveries than to those of others. Change will occur more frequently if those required to change have been involved in determining that the change is necessary.

Delineate the positive consequences that the change will have for providers and patients. Motivation to change most often occurs when events have meaning to a person. The more staff understand the purpose and process of quality assurance and the purpose of related changes that they are asked to make, the more likely they are to change.

Recognize a person's dignity and perception of a problem. People learn infrequently from authoritative sources unless they are predisposed to influence or are seeking special information. Change is more likely to occur when the people who must change believe that their motives, actions, and understanding of the issue are known and respected.

---

*Doob LW: Psychological aspects of planned developmental change. In Zaltman G, Kotler P, Kaufman I (eds): *Creating Social Change.* New York: Holt, Rinehart, Winston, 1972.

Offer opportunities for comfortable, nonthreatening peer discussions. Comfortable discussion often leads more quickly to change in concepts, values, and performance than does individual confrontation.

Apply peer pressure when appropriate. Because respected colleagues can accomplish more than a direct authority figure, peer pressure may help a person assume responsibility for his or her learning and development.

Offer opportunities for staff input into criteria development. Criteria should also be made available to staff who are being reviewed.

Provide immediate feedback on positive results of quality assurance to responsible practitioners. Such feedback reinforces staff's confidence that the value and quality of their performance is recognized.

Develop and maintain strict data security procedures that safeguard confidentiality. This reassures staff that quality assurance results are used appropriately.

Inform practitioners of deficiencies in a straightforward, nonjudgmental manner. Predictable, established mechanisms, which include safeguards for maintaining confidentiality, should be used.

Thompson and Mohr* have outlined practical issues to consider when trying to effect change, particularly when working with individual providers.

- Make certain that you are dealing with the right people, that is, the people who must change or who have the authority and power to insist upon change or who are most motivated to bring about change.
- Use a carefully thought-out, "right" approach for the person whom you are asking to change or to effect change. Select an approach that appeals to professionalism and self-interest, such as one which demonstrates without exhortation that a specific change will improve patient care and outcome.
- Confirm the facts before making a confrontation. Ascertain that you are acting on demonstrable facts rather than impressions.
- State the problem with as little value judgment as possible. For example, one might say "Here are 15 records without discharge summaries," rather than "You haven't finished your records again."
- Describe the desired behavior rather than ask for change only. Say, "When can we expect your discharge summaries and can we do anything to help?" rather than "This business of incomplete records has got to stop!"
- Have factual answers to "so whats?" Inform staff of the consequences of inappropriate actions, such as, "If discharge sum-

*Adapted from *Next Steps in Implementing Quality Appraisal Action Plans in Hospitals,* Thompson, Mohr and Associates, Oak Brook, Ill, 1980. Printed with permission.

maries are not completed within 48 hours of discharge, we are not in compliance with . . . etc, and the following actions will be taken."

- Identify, in a nonthreatening way, the monitors that will be used to measure change; for example, "Over the next six months, records for all patients whom you admit will be evaluated for completion within 72 hours of patient discharge."
- Know when to leave the issue alone for a period of time, when enough has been said to make the point, or when the issue clearly represents a "no-win" situation. In other words, the individual understands the problem, the expected change, or the consequences of no change; or the person is so resistant and defensive that further discussion will serve only to heighten antagonism.
- Provide feedback as soon as possible on the extent of change that has been made. For instance, send a letter or offer a personal comment stating, "In the past month, all but one of your records was completed in 48 hours."

Change often involves conflict, and direct confrontation is often necessary to resolve conflict. But, "people learn to avoid things that they are hit with" (Mager*), and such confrontation should be handled with care. The following suggestions on how to handle confrontation might be offered:

- Acknowledge the other person's position as legitimate.
- Differentiate the other person's position from yours.
- Determine that you understand his or her position clearly, and vice versa.
- Accept angry or hostile feelings and allow the other person to feel differently.
- Attempt to solve a problem only when the differences of opinion have been outlined completely. You know that this has occurred when you feel that you have heard, understood, and can state the differences clearly.
- Ask the other person to offer a solution and be prepared to state and differentiate yours.
- Use key phrases similar to the following during confrontation: "We see that differently." "You believe _____. On the other hand, I believe _____." "I disagree. Your position is _____; mine is _____." "Do you understand my position? It would help me if you could restate it."

---

*Mager RF: *Developing Attitude Toward Learning*. Belmont, Calif: Fearon Publishers, 1968.

Chapter 10. Evaluating and Monitoring Problem Resolution

An essential part of any quality assurance activity, reassessment is the method by which one determines and documents the extent of problem resolution. Reassessment is vital to the overall success of quality assurance activities, and should be planned and defined when corrective actions are specified. At that time, you should determine each of the following five items.

Extent of desired resolution (change). The extent of change that can logically be expected will depend on

- the state of the art of clinical practice, eg, mortality in certain diagnostic categories cannot be eradicated completely;
- the resources available in the institution, eg, staff/patient ratios might be limited by necessary financial constraints on hiring;
- the vagaries of human nature, eg, a certain percentage of physicians will always have incomplete medical records;
- the amount of change required to prevent negative impact on care if the problem continues or recurs; and
- the amount of change necessary to prevent the problem from ever recurring.

Reassessment time frame and date. The reassessment time frame should be scheduled after sufficient time has been allowed for corrective actions to have maximum effect. "Sufficient time" depends on the nature of corrective action taken. That is, the effects of change in a system (eg, additional staff, new forms, altered scheduling procedures) should be seen soon after implementation. It is likely to take longer for the effects of an extended inservice education program (eg, a three-month inservice training for nurses on education of patients undergoing renal dialysis) to become measurably apparent. Over time, these effects will vary in the extent to which they remain stable. Thus, the timing of a reassessment should be based on the type of action and an estimation of the length of time it will take to fully implement the action and to allow maximum effects of the action to occur.

Reassessment time frame and reassessment dates will differ. The reassessment time frame is the anticipated sampling period (ie, patients are selected from the past year's admissions or from admissions for the next six months, or assessment will take place over the next six months and include patients admitted in the previous six months). The reassessment date is the day or month in which a reassessment is slated to occur (ie, June 1, 1980, six months after the last inservice program).

Reassessment sample size. Generally, the reassessment sample size need not be as large as the sample reviewed in the original assessment, but it should be large enough to assess a representative portion of care and to determine the extent of resolution. In situations in which staff suspect that a problem persists but reassessment does not confirm that judgment, the reassessment sample size may have been too small. In some of these instances, the reassessment sample may have to be larger than the sample used for the initial assessment. (For further discussion of sampling techniques, see Chapter 8.)

Responsibility for reassessment. The individuals who are responsible for implementing the reassessment activity should be identified, and their duties should be specified clearly.

Method of reassessment. The method of reassessment need not be the same method or on the same scale as the original assessment. For example, a reassessment monitor for actions taken as the result of a full-scale audit might entail the use of one criterion only. Or, direct observation of actual patient education activities might replace review of a large sample of patient education flow charts from the original assessment.

Lack of Problem Resolution

When reassessment activity indicates that the problem has not been corrected, review initial assessment results and subsequent events to determine whether

- the site and nature of the problem and the audience for intervention were correctly determined;
- identified corrective actions were appropriate to the site and nature of the problem and to the audience;
- actions were feasible;
- authority and responsibility for implementing actions were specified clearly and correctly;
- actions were indeed implemented; and
- reassessment sample size was adequate.

Should you identify errors in any one or combination of these areas, it might be necessary to reconstruct appropriate, feasible corrective actions; to redefine authority and responsibility for implementing those actions; and to monitor the implementation and impact of the corrective actions. On the other hand, if deficiencies occurred in none of these areas, the problem may not have been corrected because of adamant resistance to change. Should this be the case, it may be necessary simply to monitor the problem so that it does not increase in magnitude and attempt resolution at a later date, after methods to decrease resistance, such as those outlined in Chapters 5 and 9, have been applied.

Chapter 11. Evaluating a Quality Assurance Program

Your quality assurance program can only be effective if each part is performed at its maximum level. Both the quality assurance program as a whole and the individual quality assurance activities should be evaluated. Annual and periodic evaluation should assist you in determining whether the goals and objectives of the program are being met; whether strengths in the program are being maintained and weaknesses corrected; and whether the program and its activities are keeping pace with the evolution of standards and regulations, and with advances in medical and scientific practice and technology. To comply with JCAH quality assurance requirements, the quality assurance program should be evaluated at least annually. At the outset, however, you might wish to evaluate the quality assurance program more often so that the effectiveness of change can be determined.

Responsibility for evaluating the quality assurance program should be specified in the hospital's quality assurance plan. Actual assessment of the quality assurance program and activities can be delegated to the committees and departments that conduct quality assurance activities or to a quality assurance department. Analysis of the assessment and/or approval of any recommended modifications or alterations in the program should be accomplished by those with authority and responsibility for the overall quality assurance program.

Evaluation Questions

Although the questions which follow are designed to assist you to evaluate your quality assurance program on an annual or periodic basis, they might also prove useful in evaluating your current program. They can be used separately from or in addition to the assessment questions that appear in Chapter 2.

Organization

The following questions are relevant to evaluating the organization of the quality assurance program.

- Are all disciplines that provide patient care represented in quality assurance activities?
- Are all medical staff review requirements met?
- Are all nursing and support services review and evaluation requirements met?
- Are hospital-wide review requirements met?
- Are the governing body and administration actively involved in the program? That is, do they receive regular reports and/or are they active members of a committee responsible for corrective action?
- Does each committee chairperson understand the function of his or her committee and any related committees?
- Do all departments have a demonstrable understanding of the definition and application of quality assurance? Can they identify ongoing quality assurance committees and functions? Do they understand their roles and what is required of them?
- Is the administration/coordination of the overall quality assurance program accomplished effectively and efficiently?
- Can coordination be improved and activities integrated further to provide for more effective use of resources?

Problem-Focused Approach

The following questions are relevant to the process of problem identification and resolution.

- Are important and meaningful problems (those which may have a negative impact on patient care if not resolved) identified?
- Are there additional data sources that could be used to identify problems?
- Are priorities set equitably?
- Are priorities updated periodically?
- If priorities are not set centrally within the hospital but are set on a departmental basis, is there a mechanism for central review and approval?
- Are identified problems assessed to determine cause and scope?
- Are predetermined, clinically valid criteria used to identify and assess problems?

- Are the appropriate individuals responsible for implementing action?
- Are recommended actions frequently not implemented?
- What problems have not been resolved? Why?
- Are problems monitored to determine if they are resolved or reduced to an acceptable level?
- Are problems monitored by the appropriate individuals?

Reporting

Investigate the potential for reporting on quality assurance activities through the following series of questions.

- Does each quality assurance function report to the appropriate and designated individuals, groups, or committees?
- Is the frequency of reporting adequate?
- Is the method (eg, committee minutes) used to report findings effective?
- Is quality assurance information used in medical staff reappraisals and hospital staff performance appraisals?
- Is evaluation of the performance of the hospital administrator and chiefs of service based in part on the accomplishments of quality assurance activities?
- Has quality assurance information been used to plan education activities (eg, continuing education, inservice programs, orientation)?
- Is there a system for regular input of quality assurance information to the group responsible for resource allocation (ie, manpower/personnel planning, equipment committee, budget) and to short-range and long-range planning efforts?

Impact

Finally, the following questions should be raised to identify areas in which improvements in patient care/clinical performance have been made or areas in which evaluation efforts need to be focused.

- How do outcome indicators such as morbidity/mortality, infection, and complication rates or LOS compare with previous measures?
- Did the results of the activities improve patient care? How?
- Did the results of the activities improve clinical performance? How?
- Is the program/activity cost-effective?
- What changes should be implemented to improve the quality assurance program?
- What new objectives should be set?

Appendix A.
Case Study Exercises

The case studies provided in this appendix illustrate approaches to planning quality assurance (QA) programs that were developed in actual hospital facilities—a small rural hospital (Hospital A); a medium-sized rural hospital (Hospital B); an urban community hospital (Hospital C); a community teaching hospital (Hospital D); and a university affiliated hospital (Hospital E).

The case studies demonstrate how these hospitals assessed their QA activities in 1979, analyzed the strengths and weaknesses of those activities, and developed proposed QA plans that would help them organize an integrated, coordinated QA program. An outline of the hospital's quality assurance activities in 1979 and of the proposed quality assurance plan is included for each of the case studies provided in this appendix. The plans are published for illustrative purposes only and do not necessarily reflect compliance with QA requirements of JCAH. The responsibility for developing a QA plan lies with each hospital.

Hospital A: Small Rural Hospital

A 68-bed, rural, acute-care general hospital, Hospital A is the only hospital serving a population of 33,000 in two counties. The services provided are primarily medical and surgical, although the hospital has a coronary care unit, emergency room, physical and respiratory therapy departments, and an outpatient department. Primary health care services are provided at two satellite facilities.

The governing body consists of four trustees appointed by the county commissioners. The five general practitioners and one family practitioner who comprise the full-time medical staff are complemented by 20 specialists on the consultant and courtesy staff.

Quality Assurance Activities in 1979

The governing body delegates responsibility for quality assurance to the medical staff through the chief executive officer (CEO). A QA coordinator (nonphysician) has been appointed to oversee the QA plan, which consists of utilization review and medical audit. An assistant to the coordinator helps with data retrieval.

Two committees of the active medical staff are responsible, respectively, for utilization review and medical audit. The medical audit committee is also responsible for tissue review, infection control, pharmacy and therapeutics, blood transfusion review, and risk management activities. Audit results are presented to the entire medical staff. The medical staff and CEO support the audit function, and the governing body shows interest in study results.

Analysis of the Assessment Matrix

Because the administrator, assistant administrator, and QA coordinator attend all medical staff meetings, communication about QA activities is readily facilitated. Proposed changes in the current QA program will emphasize integration of all functions that have an impact on the quality of patient care. Emphasis on medical audit as the sole measure of quality of care will be expanded to include other functions as well. (See the completed assessment matrix on page 137.)

Medical Staff Organization, Hospital A

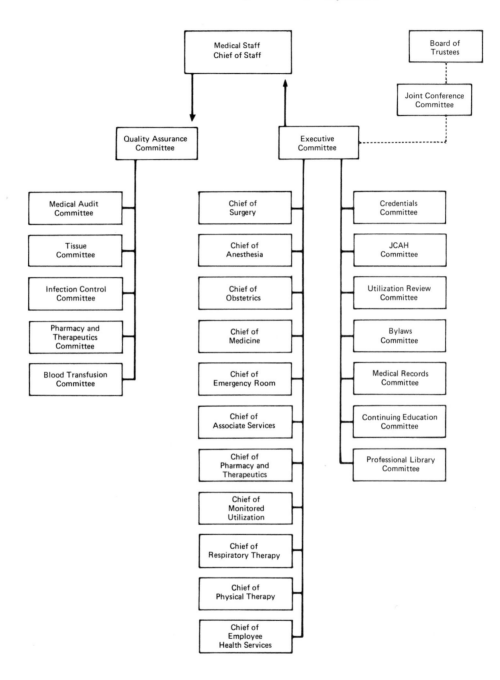

Current Organizational Chart, Hospital A

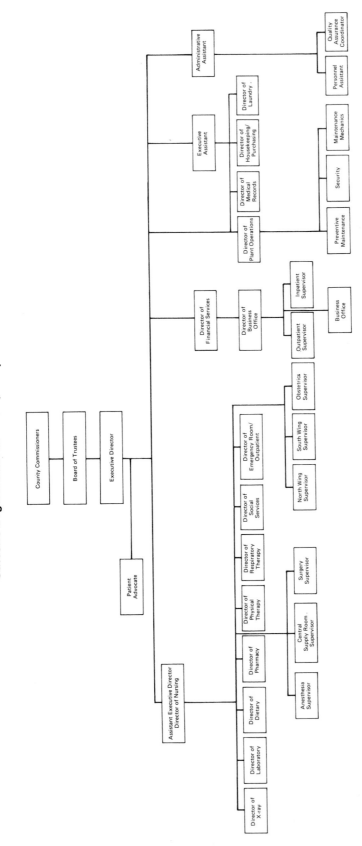

Completed Assessment Matrix, Hospital A

Assessment Questions	Credentialing	Clinical Department Review	Tissue/Surgical Case Review and Evaluation	Morbidity/Mortality	Pharmacy and Therapeutics	Blood Utilization Review and Evaluation	Antibiotic Usage Review and Evaluation	Nursing Care Review and Evaluation	Review and Evaluation of Support Services	Audit	Infection Control	Safety	Utilization Review	Risk Control	Continuing Education	Accreditation	Patient Representative Information
1. Is the function performed by an individual or committee?	C	Both	C	C	C	C	C	C	C	C	Both	C	Both	C	C	No	—
2. Who is routinely responsible for the function?	CS	Dept head	Chairman	Chairman	Chairman	Chairman	Pharmacy	Nursing director	Chairman	Chairman	IC nurse	Chairman	UR coordinator	Chairman	CS		—
3. Is there a written description or procedure for the function?	Yes	Not all	Yes	Yes	Yes	Yes	Yes	Yes	Yes	Yes	Yes	Yes	Yes	?	Yes		
4. What data sources are used to perform this function?	Applications, references	Various	MRs, TRs	?	Education, MRs, TRs	MRs, lab reports	?	MRs	MRs	MRs	MRs, lab reports	Incident reports	MRs	Incident reports, med error	Audit results		Direct patient contact
5. Are preestablished, clinically valid criteria used?	Yes	Yes	?	?	?	?	?	Yes	Yes	Yes	Yes	Yes	Yes	?	No		No
6. If a purpose of the function is to identify problems, are important problems identified?	Yes	No	Yes	?	Yes	Yes	Yes	Yes	Yes	Yes	Yes	?	No	?	Yes		Yes
7. Does the responsible individual or committee recommend or implement action?	R	Both	R	R	R	R	R	Both	R	R	R	R	Both	R	Both		?
8. Is there monitoring to determine effectiveness of action?	No	Yes	No	?	?	?	?	Yes	?	Yes	Yes	?	Yes	?	No		R
9. To whom are the results of the function reported? With whom are they shared?	Board	?	MEC	MEC	MEC	MEC	MEC	MS, board	?	CS, MEC	MEC	MEC	MEC	CEO	MS	CEO	No
10. Is the function evaluated routinely?	?	Yes	?	?	?	?	?	No	?	?	?	?	?	?	?	?	?

C=committee
CEO=chief executive officer
CS=chief of staff
I=individual
IC=infection control

MEC=medical executive committee
MR=medical record
MS=medical staff
OR=operating room
R=recommends

TR=tissue reports
UR=utilization review
?=do not know

Proposed Quality Assurance Plan for Hospital A

Rationale. The QA program at Hospital A is designed to maintain and improve the quality of patient care throughout the hospital with the best utilization of scarce resources.

At Hospital A, quality assurance is defined as the integration of quality assessment and quality control activities throughout the hospital to maintain and/or raise the standard of care. Every activity throughout the hospital that has an impact on the quality of care will be monitored by the QA committee.

Previously, methods for controlling quality of care have functioned autonomously. Addressing quality assurance from an overall perspective and integrating existing QA activities is intended to provide another dimension of quality. Centralizing the QA program will clarify responsibility and accountability.

To implement the new JCAH standard on quality assurance, we have taken all elements in the hospital that have impact on the quality of care and have clarified their interrelationships. The decision to capitalize on existing mechanisms was determined to be most effective in minimizing duplication, disruptive change, and additional work.

Objectives. QA activities throughout the hospital will be integrated by the QA committee. Each department or function that has an impact on patient care will be outlined on the QA organizational chart (see the opposite page), and the reporting mechanism for quality of care activities will be identified. Each function (department, committee, process, individual) will outline goals and objectives to identify and resolve problems related to the quality of care. Goals and objectives will reflect how problems are to be identified, analyzed, and corrected. Quality of care will be viewed from a problem/action/result model. Minutes of meetings will describe results. Minutes will reflect the problem/action/result model and will be identified in a separate section on quality assurance in the minutes of all committees.

Organization. The QA plan will be implemented by the QA coordinator who will disseminate written guidelines to each function identified on the organizational chart. These written guidelines will clarify what quality assurance is and identify each function's QA responsibility.

The QA coordinator will coordinate all QA activities with the QA committee and the assistant executive director, and will attend meetings of all QA functions.

Minutes of all QA activities will be sent to the QA committee for action by the chief of staff (for physician-related problems) or by the assistant executive director and the QA coordinator (for all nonphysician-related problems). Follow-up reports will be given to each committee.

Evaluation. The QA coordinator will compile all problems/actions/results identified by each function on an annual basis. The QA committee will determine the effectiveness of the efforts and will identify changes for the committees, medical staff, and administration.

Functional Organization of Proposed Quality Assurance Plan, Hospital A

Hospital B: Medium-Sized Rural Hospital

Hospital B is a 118-bed, multilevel health care facility located in the rural south-central area of the United States. A not-for-profit community hospital that is approximately 28 years old, Hospital B has added a hospital-based, skilled nursing facility and a personal care facility to its services within the past 10 years. The hospital was founded to provide care to the people of the community and to World War II veterans who live in the county. As the only health care facility in the county, Hospital B provides services to an agricultural and small industrial community/population of 15,000. Approximately 2,400 patients are admitted to the facility annually. A 95% average occupancy rate is maintained in the two long term care units. Hospital B is licensed and certified by the state department of health and appropriate federal agencies (Medicare and Medical Assistance) and has consistently received a two-year accreditation from the Joint Commission on Accreditation of Hospitals.

A governing body appointed by the fiscal court has ultimate responsibility for the overall management and operation of the facility. The chairman of the governing body is elected by its members. The CEO is employed by the governing body to act on its behalf and has served in his present position for the past nine years. Prior to his employment, the CEO was a member of the governing body. The governing body delegates authority to the medical staff for the review and evaluation of medical care and other medical staff functions within the facility. The medical staff is organized as a committee of the whole and is nondepartmentalized. This approach is effective because of the size of the institution and the scope of medical services provided.

Quality Assurance Activities in 1979

The commitment and attitudes of the governing body, medical staff, administration, and individual support services toward QA activities performed within the institution have been most positive. A multidisciplinary approach to audit (patient care evaluation) was used for five years, and no significant interferences or problems were encountered with this approach. During the past year, a "problem-focused approach" to evaluation has been used, and this approach has been more effective than audits conducted on diagnoses or procedures.

Each support service has responsibility for the regular review and evaluation of its activities. Presently, findings from support services review are presented to the medical staff by the QA coordinator at its scheduled meetings. To date, however, each support service conducts review without communication with other support services that might also be involved. A more integrated approach to review and evaluation by hospital support services would enhance the overall hospital program.

Analysis of the Assessment Matrix

QA activities at Hospital B are operational, function efficiently, and are fairly effective (see the completed matrix on the opposite page). Little or no duplication of activities exists, and sufficient time and resources are allocated for QA activities.

Integration of activities can be enhanced, however, particularly in the area of support services review and evaluation. Integration of medical and nursing staff activities already exists, but analysis and planning follow-up can be improved.

Completed Assessment Matrix, Hospital B

Assessment Questions	Credentialing	Clinical Department Review	Tissue/Surgical Case Review and Evaluation	Morbidity/Mortality	Pharmacy and Therapeutics	Blood Utilization Review and Evaluation	Antibiotic Usage Review and Evaluation	Nursing Care Review and Evaluation	Review and Evaluation of Support Services	Audit	Infection Control	Safety	Utilization Review	Risk Control	Continuing Education	Accreditation	Patient Representative Information
1. Is the function performed by an individual or committee?	C	C	C	C	C	C	C	C	Individual service	C	C	C	C	I	I	I	I
2. Who is routinely responsible for the function?	Chairman		Chairman	Chairman	Chairman	Chairman	ICC	Nursing admin	Dept head	Chairman	Chairman	Safety director	Chairman	Admin	Staff dev coord	Admin, MS	Admin
3. Is there a written description or procedure for the function?	Yes	Yes	Yes	No	Yes	Yes	Yes	Yes	Yes	Yes	Yes	Yes	Yes	No	Yes	Yes	Yes
4. What data sources are used to perform this function?	References		MRs, OR	MRs	antibiotic review	MRs, lab	ICC files, MRs, pharmacy	NRs, MRs, IRs	NRs, MRs, IRs	MRs, IR	Lab, isolation files	MRs, IRs	MRs	IRs, PI	Audit results & others	JCAH reports	PI
5. Are preestablished, clinically valid criteria used?	No	Yes	Yes	No	?	Yes	Yes	Yes	Yes	Yes	Yes	Yes	?	No	No	?	No
6. If a purpose of the function is to identify problems, are important problems identified?	Yes	Yes	Yes	No	Yes	Yes	Yes	Yes	Yes	Yes	Yes	Yes	Yes	Yes	Yes	Yes	Yes
7. Does the responsible individual or committee recommend or implement action?	R	IA	IA	IA	IA	IA	IA	IA	IA	R	R	R	IA	IA	R	IA	R
8. Is there monitoring to determine effectiveness of action?	Yes	Yes	Yes	Yes	Yes	Yes	Yes	Yes	Yes	Yes	Yes	Yes	Yes	Yes	Yes	Yes	Yes
9. To whom are the results of the function reported? With whom are they shared?	?	?	?	?	?	?	?	?	?	?	?	?	?	?	?	?	?
10. Is the function evaluated routinely?	Yes	Yes	Yes	Yes	Yes	Yes	Yes	Yes	Yes	Yes	Yes	Yes	Yes	Yes	Yes	Yes	Yes

C=committee
I=individual
IA=implements action
ICC=infection control committee
IR=incident report
MR=medical record
MS=medical staff
NR=nursing record
OR=operating room
PI=patient interview
R=recommends
?=do not know

Proposed Quality Assurance Plan for Hospital B

Purpose. The governing body, medical staff, and professional service staff of Hospital B will demonstrate a consistent endeavor to deliver patient care that is optimal within available resources and is consistent with achievable goals for the institution.

Goals. Hospital B's QA program will establish, maintain, support, and document evidence of an ongoing QA program that includes effective mechanisms for reviewing and evaluating patient care and for appropriate response to findings, and will establish priorities for problem resolution by focusing on the resolution of known or suspected problems that have a direct or indirect impact on patients and/or by focusing on areas with potential for substantial improvements in patient care.

Objectives. The governing body and the CEO will support QA activities within the institution by assuming responsibility for the ongoing QA program; by providing administrative staff to assist in review functions; and by acting on findings/recommendations related to action implemented to sustain resolution of problems. The medical staff will define the scope of quality assessment activities to be monitored and will determine the mechanism and type of review function to be performed (prospective, concurrent, retrospective). As specified in the plan, each clinical discipline (professional staff) will participate in the review of the patient care it provides. Results/findings will be communicated to the appropriate bodies. When possible, professional staffs will perform review functions/activities with the medical staff. QA activities will be integrated, coordinated, cost-effective, consistent, and designed to minimize duplication of effort.

Outline of the Scope of Proposed Quality Assurance Activities

I. Medical Staff Review Functions
    A. Reappointment and credentialing
    B. Utilization review
    C. Patient care evaluation studies
    D. Clinical monitors
        1. Blood utilization
        2. Tissue review
        3. Mortality review
        4. Antibiotic review
        5. Review of pharmacy and therapeutics committee functions
        6. Other patient related activities (eg, infection control and safety committees)
    E. Continuing medical education
II. Other Professional Staffs Review Functions
    A. Each clinical discipline will be responsible for identifying and resolving problems related to the patient care they provide. Findings

related to quality of care provided by a clinical unit that is not represented in a specific assessment activity will be made available to the director of the unit.

B. Findings of QA activities throughout the hospital shall be reported to the QA coordinator, the medical staff, the CEO, and the governing body.

C. The following disciplines/services participate in quality assessment activities.
1. Anesthesia
2. Dietary
3. Emergency
4. Nursing
5. Pathology and medical laboratory
6. Pharmacy
7. Radiology
8. Rehabilitation
9. Respiratory care
10. Social service

Organizational Plan

Authority. The governing body will have final authority and responsibility for the assurance of a flexible, comprehensive, and integrated QA program. It will have the responsibility for assuring the public of optimal quality of all care delivered by professionals within the institution. The governing body delegates authority and accountability for the operation of the program to the medical staff. Other staff professionals are delegated the responsibility for the delivery and evaluation of the care they provide through their clinical services.

The governing body and hospital administration will assume responsibility for assuring that the QA program is specifically compatible with requirements of third-party payers, including federal and state governments. The governing body will make the commitment to provide the financial support necessary for the QA program so that administration can provide the specific resources in service, equipment, and personnel required; and it will make all final determinations of the extent, if any, to which outside aids (consultants, voluntary or mandatory review bodies) will be used in QA activities to identify and/or assess problems.

The governing body will receive reports through the appropriate organizational plan of the findings of QA activities.

Functions. The medical staff will make the commitment to actively participate in and manage the QA program. The medical staff is delegated authority and accountability for the delivery and evaluation of medical functions and activities. The medical staff will also define the scope of QA activities to be performed; develop preestablished criteria to be utilized as a screening mechanism; review findings of QA activities;

identify/assess problems; plan/monitor corrective action; and report findings to the governing body.

The QA coordinator will attend all medical staff committee meetings in which monitoring functions or QA activities are performed, and utilize preestablished screening criteria to prepare data for review/evaluation functions of the medical staff. These functions include, but are not limited to, blood utilization, tissue review, mortality, and medical records.

Other functions performed by the QA coordinator include:

- assisting the secretary to the medical staff and the director of nursing to maintain committee meetings concerned with QA activities;
- assisting medical, nursing, and other professional staffs in the development of written criteria used to assess problems when necessary, as well as providing references, criteria developed in outside organizations, or model criteria sets;
- promoting consistency in QA activities by developing a source of definitions for terminology used to describe studies performed or methods employed; and
- assisting in integration of QA activities between medical, nursing, and other professional staffs.

The nursing service staff will participate in the regular review and evaluation of the quality of care they provide, and will develop preestablished criteria for use in evaluation. Where possible, nursing service evaluation activities should be integrated with the evaluation activities of the medical staff. Evaluation activities will be coordinated through the QA coordinator. Findings will be reported to the CEO, the medical staff, and others when appropriate.

Other professional staff will evaluate the quality of care they provide. Each service will establish criteria to monitor its practice. When possible, evaluation activities of each service will be coordinated with the evaluation activities of the medical, nursing, and other professional staffs. Again, evaluation activities will be coordinated through the QA coordinator.

Evaluation. The governing body and the medical staff committee of the whole will appraise the QA plan at least annually to assure that the collective effort is comprehensive and cost-effective, shows minimal duplication of effort, and results in improved patient care. The appraisal will identify components of the QA program that need to be instituted, altered, or deleted.

Proposed Quality Assurance Chart, Hospital B

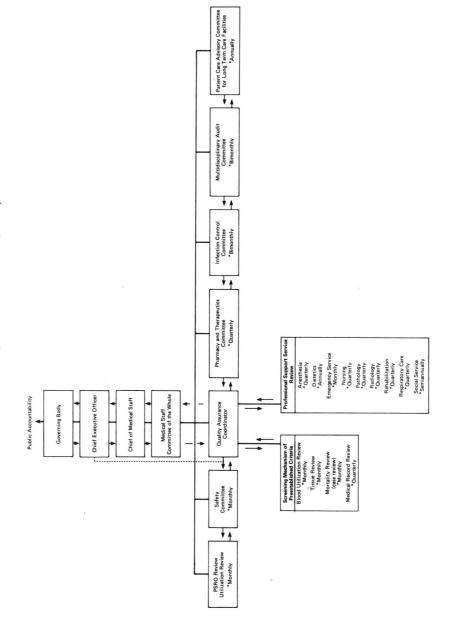

Hospital C: Urban Community Hospital

Founded in 1886, Hospital C is a 251-bed, voluntary, not-for-profit general medical and surgical hospital located in a densely populated urban area. According to the 1970 census, Hospital C serves approximately 91,000 people with a broad mix of socioeconomic, racial, and ethnic characteristics. Projections for 1985 predict that the population will increase by at least 16%.

In addition to a medical staff of over 200 physicians, the hospital has 640 full-time and 75 part-time employees. Physicians on the medical staff represent 24 medical and surgical specialties; approximately 80% are board certified, and many hold faculty appointments at medical schools and university hospitals.

Hospital C has an emergency department that provides coverage by a licensed physician 24 hours a day, seven days a week. Physicians who represent major specialties are on call within minutes. The surgical department performs an average of 12 surgical procedures daily. The hospital laboratory provides a full range of biologic, bacteriologic, and chemical tests. The department of radiology provides all major diagnostic x-ray examinations and nuclear medicine studies. The physical therapy department provides hydrotherapy, electrotherapy, rehabilitation, and a recently instituted program for pain management and control. The department also offers extensive rehabilitation programs for patients who have experienced stroke, amputation, burns, and orthopedic and chest surgery. Speech therapy is also available.

The respiratory therapy department provides tests and treatment for all chronic pulmonary diseases. The social service department locates rehabilitation facilities and specialized care, as well as home health care, home delivered meals, and home management after hospital discharge for patients with chronic and long-term illnesses. A fully staffed outpatient department provides services from 8:00 AM to 4:00 PM, Monday through Saturday. A complete electroencephalographic laboratory, an electromyographic nerve conduction laboratory, and a cardiographic department were opened in 1977. The hospital recently completed construction of an examining room for EENT and dental patients.

Hospital C provides a student rotation for junior and senior students in podiatry. The hospital maintains around-the-clock housestaff coverage in both medicine and surgery by qualified licensed physicians who have completed postgraduate training.

Quality Assurance Activities in 1979

Primary responsibility for the QA program is vested in the board of directors. The board, through the president of the hospital, delegates authority for direction of the QA program to the medical director and medical staff. The medical staff, in turn, delegates operational authority to several standing committees (see Current Organizational Chart, Hospital C, page 152), including the quality care and audit committee.

Quality care and audit committee. Although members change on an annual basis, the quality care and audit committee always includes representatives of each medical service and of the clinical pathology, radiology, nursing, social services, and medical record departments. Representatives from physical and respiratory therapy, dietary services, and the pharmacy are invited to participate in meetings at which audits that touch on their areas of patient care are planned or reviewed. The medical director and the associate director of medical education serve as ex officio members with full voting rights.

Structure of the patient care evaluation program. During the early years of QA activities at Hospital C, the quality care and audit committee based its choice of audit topics on the incidence of various diagnoses and procedures found in discharge statistics. In the past two years, however, the committee increasingly has chosen audit topics based on perceived problems in care, morbidity, and recommendations from the patient care committee.

The patient care committee, composed of representatives from all hospital disciplines, acts as a forum for problems in patient care. This committee takes action on certain problems and recommends serious problems to the quality care and audit committee for further study.

QA activities are based on the medical staff bylaws and rules and regulations, dated March 1974. The administration and medical staff of Hospital C are committed to the concept of quality assurance, although the medical staff approaches quality assurance in a much less structured manner.

In the present system, most recommendations are referred to the medical executive committee. Matters of great importance to the medical staff are handled, but matters of less direct consequence to the medical staff tend to "fall between the cracks." In addition, the basic political nature of the medical executive committee sometimes interferes with the current QA effort because it is poorly defined (see the illustration shown below of the current relationship among administration, medical staff, and governing body).

Current Relationship Among Administration, Medical Staff, and Governing Body, Hospital C

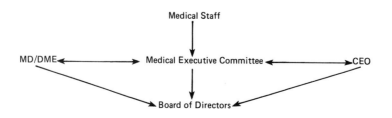

Analysis of the Assessment Matrix

Using the completed assessment matrix on page 153, Hospital C staff identified the following problems in their QA program:

- limited knowledge about the extent of and responsibility for risk control activities in the hospital;
- limited knowledge about the extent and impact of support services evaluation activities;
- committees require assistance in writing criteria and identifying topics for study;
- priorities for problem-solving have not been set;
- committees recommend actions to the medical executive committee, but recommendations do not go beyond that committee;
- authority for implementing actions is lacking;
- feedback mechanisms need to be improved;
- communications need to be centralized and formalized;
- routine follow-up of actions is difficult;
- bylaws need to be reexamined; and
- QA activities require integration.

Current Organizational Chart, Hospital C

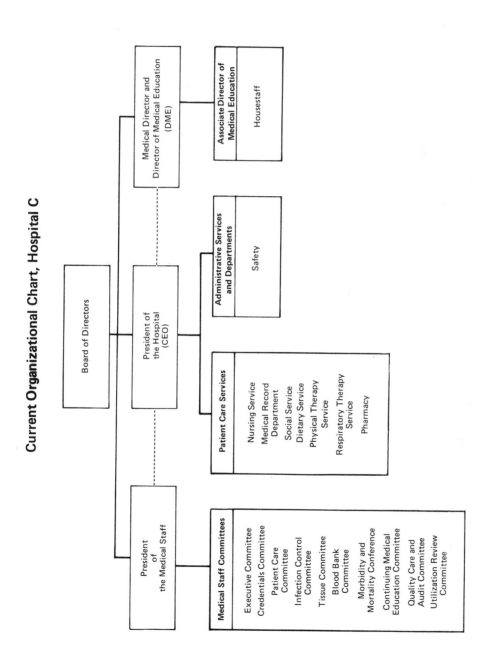

Completed Assessment Matrix, Hospital C

Assessment Questions	Credentialing	Clinical Department Review	Tissue/Surgical Case Review and Evaluation	Morbidity/Mortality	Pharmacy and Therapeutics	Blood Utilization Review and Evaluation	Antibiotic Usage Review and Evaluation	Nursing Care Review and Evaluation	Review and Evaluation of Support Services	Audit	Infection Control	Safety	Utilization Review	Risk Control	Continuing Education	Accreditation	Patient Representative Information
1. Is the function performed by an individual or committee?	C	I	C	C	C	C	C	C	?	C	Both	C	Both	?	Both	C	Both
2. Who is routinely responsible for the function?	Med director	Dept head	MD, pathologist	MD, med director	MD, Chairman	MD, pathologist	MD, chairman	Chairman	?	Chairman	MD, chairman	EVP	RN/MD	EVP	DME	MD, chairman	Nursing director
3. Is there a written description or procedure for the function?	Yes	No	Yes	No	Yes	Yes	?	Yes	?	Yes	Yes	Yes	Yes	No	No	Yes	No
4. What data sources are used to perform this function?	Interviews, references	Various	MRs, PRs	MRs, PRs	Pharmacy logs	?	?	MRs	?	MRs	MRs, Lab reports	IRs	MRs	IRs	Audit results & surveys	JCAH standards	Patient contact
5. Are preestablished, clinically valid criteria used?	Yes	Occasionally	Yes	No	No	Yes	Yes	Yes	?	Yes	?	Yes	Yes	No	NA	Yes	NA
6. If a purpose of the function is to identify problems, are important problems identified?	Yes	Yes / Occa-sionally	Yes	Yes	Yes	Yes	Yes	Yes	?	Yes	Yes	Yes	Yes	Yes	Yes	Yes	Yes
7. Does the responsible individual or committee recommend or implement action?	Both	Both	R	R	R	R	R	R	R	Both	R	R	Both	R	Both	Both	Both
8. Is there monitoring to determine effectiveness of action?	Yes	Occasionally	Yes	Yes	?	Yes	Yes	Yes	?	Yes	Yes	Yes	Yes	?	Yes	Yes	Yes
9. To whom are the results of the function reported? With whom are they shared?	MEC, board	Admin	MEC	MEC	MEC, pharmacy	MEC	MEC	MEC	?	MEC, staff	MEC, lab	Admin	MEC	Admin	MEC	Board	EVP
10. Is the function evaluated routinely?	?	No	?	?	?	?	?	?	?	?	?	?	?	?	?	?	?

C=committee
EVP=executive vice president
DME=director of medical education
IR=incident report
MEC=medical executive committee

MR=medical record
OR=operating room
PR=pathology report
R=recommends
?=do not know

Proposed Quality Assurance Plan for Hospital C

Goal. The goal of the QA program is to restore patients to the highest levels of health and well-being that are possible within available resources.

Purpose. The purpose of Hospital C's QA program is to prevent premature mortality and unnecessary morbidity and its attendant discomfort, disease, deformity, disability, and expense for patients, the hospital and medical staffs, visitors, and the surrounding community. The QA program should be cost-effective and time-efficient (process), without sacrificing the quality of patient care reflected in better health (outcome).

Objective. The objective of the program is to reduce and/or eliminate unnecessary and correctable risks, hazards, and expense within the hospital through:

- establishing an ongoing monitor for problem identification;
- objectively assessing the cause and scope of identified problems;
- establishing priorities for the resolution of identified problems;
- implementing appropriate mechanisms for problem-solving;
- assuring that corrective action is appropriate and sustained through ongoing follow-up of problem-solving activities; and
- documenting improved patient care and improved patient outcome through QA efforts.

Organization

Quality assurance board. The QA plan will establish a QA board that will be composed of the following:

- the QA coordinator, who will be responsible for meeting agendas and for the day-to-day functioning of the QA program;
- the CEO or a designee;
- the medical director or a designee;
- representatives from the medical executive committee, such as the president of the medical staff;
- a major department head, such as the vice-president of nursing; and
- consultants as needed to review particular problems.

The QA board will perform the following functions:

- meet regularly (eg, on a weekly basis) or at any time that an urgent situation warrants a meeting;
- coordinate problem identification;
- establish priorities;
- delegate responsibilities for problem-solving;
- follow-up for corrective action; and
- monitor regularly (eg, on a quarterly basis) to ensure that problems remain corrected.

Authority for the QA board will be vested through the bylaws of the hospital, the medical staff, and the board of directors.

Accountability of the QA board will ultimately be to the patient population served. Nevertheless, the QA board will be directly accountable to the board of directors, which will review the QA program on an annual basis for evidence of improved patient care, achievement of goals and objectives, and cost-effectiveness.

Quality assurance activities. Each QA activity will follow the procedure outlined in the Implementation Flow Chart (shown below) by identifying and evaluating problems and reporting findings to the QA board.

The tissue committee will refer to the QA board all surgical procedures defined as follows in Section VI, Part B, subsection 3.4, Medical Staff Bylaws: "The preoperative diagnosis and surgical findings are not appropriately interrelated, and from the record, it appears that surgery was not justified."

The blood bank committee will refer inappropriate utilization of blood products and complications resulting therefrom to the QA board.

Implementation Flow Chart for Each QA Function, Hospital C

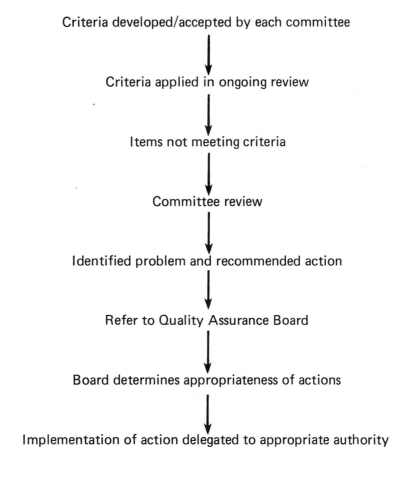

Criteria developed/accepted by each committee

↓

Criteria applied in ongoing review

↓

Items not meeting criteria

↓

Committee review

↓

Identified problem and recommended action

↓

Refer to Quality Assurance Board

↓

Board determines appropriateness of actions

↓

Implementation of action delegated to appropriate authority

The UR committee will report significant variations from the standard length of stay criteria to the QA board. It should also refer overutilization or underutilization of hospital services to the QA board.

The infection control committee will refer significant variations of antibiotic usage to the QA board. The committee should also report significant patterns of infections, contamination, and iatrogenic and nosocomial infections.

The pharmacy and therapeutics committee will report significant variations in medication usage to the QA board. It will also refer complications of drug therapy and drug interactions as defined by a patient's compatibility profile.

The patient care committee will refer relevant patient care items obtained from patient surveys or patient representatives (nursing supervisors, the vice-president of marketing, social service department) to the QA board.

The disaster and emergency department will refer significant items relating to patient care in the areas of physician and support service response time and appropriate disposition and follow-up of emergency room patients to the QA board.

The continuing medical education (CME) committee will document and report the effectiveness of the CME program in improving patient care to the QA board.

The mortality and morbidity conference will refer significant mortality findings identified in its monthly review activity to the QA board.

Risk control will report significant information relating to medical staff performance in the areas of patterns of complications, lawsuits, and patient complaints to the credentials and privileges committee.

Particular attention will be paid to cost-effectiveness of testing and to effective coordination of various hospital staffs involved in patient care, including discharge planning information and problems identified by the social service.

Evaluation. Each function shall be responsible for ongoing evaluation and annual assessment of specific goals and objectives and for reporting such evaluation to the QA board.

Proposed Quality Assurance Organizational Chart, Hospital C

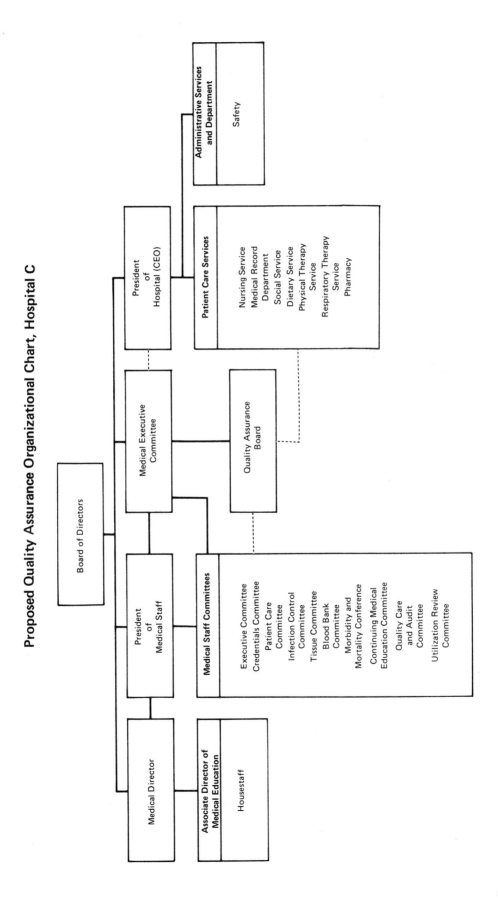

Hospital D: Community Teaching Hospital

A 500-bed acute care community teaching institution, Hospital D has 1,800 employees and over 100 residents and interns in training. The hospital has approximately 21,000 admissions per year and maintains a 90% average occupancy rate. Specialized services that are often found in larger university teaching centers are available, including a physical and rehabilitative medicine center; an active inpatient and outpatient psychiatric department; a research center and animal laboratory; and student training programs in respiratory and physical therapy, radiologic technology, and various levels of nursing. The intensive care neonatology and high-risk obstetrical centers offer specialized treatment for pregnant women and newborn children.

Hospital D is governed by a board of directors. Day-to-day responsibility for the operation of the institution is delegated to the executive vice-president and executed through a group of vice-presidents. The medical departments are headed by full-time chiefs of service, each of whom is responsible for the day-to-day operation and quality of their divisions. A medical executive committee, composed of the full-time chiefs of service and attending physicians, recommends medical policy to the board of directors on behalf of the medical staff. The medical staff has its own officers and members—almost 700 individual practitioners in 12 departments. Over 100 of these physicians are full-time hospital employees.

Quality Assurance Activities in 1979

The overall responsibility for the QA program lies with the board of directors. Responsibility for implementation is delegated to the medical staff and its committees. Certain required quality review activities take place through a series of committees and are filtered through a single QA committee that is ultimately responsible to the medical staff and the board of directors. Representatives of nursing service administration and the medical staff sit on the various committees. Utilization review coordinators help staff with medical audit, utilization review, and medical record review.

Only four committees report through the single QA committee to the board (the tissue review, medical records, utilization review, and audit committees). However, as many as ten other committees with responsibilities in quality assurance are not coordinated by a single activity, but report to the medical executive committee (see current Quality Assurance Organizational Chart, page 161). The existing QA program has several problems that must be addressed so that optimum quality of care within the institution can be assured.

Analysis of the Assessment Matrix

Using the completed assessment matrix on page 162, Hospital D staff identified the following problems in their quality assurance program:

- duplication of effort exists among various quality assurance activities;
- establishment of priorities for problem-solving is not coordinated by one central committee;
- coordination of problem identification/resolution is lacking;
- a central committee that acts as a clearinghouse for results/findings is lacking;
- appropriate follow-up is not guaranteed;
- although staffing for QA activities is adequate, staff are not allocated where most needed; and
- predetermined measurable criteria are not always used when appropriate.

Current Quality Assurance Organizational Chart, Hospital D

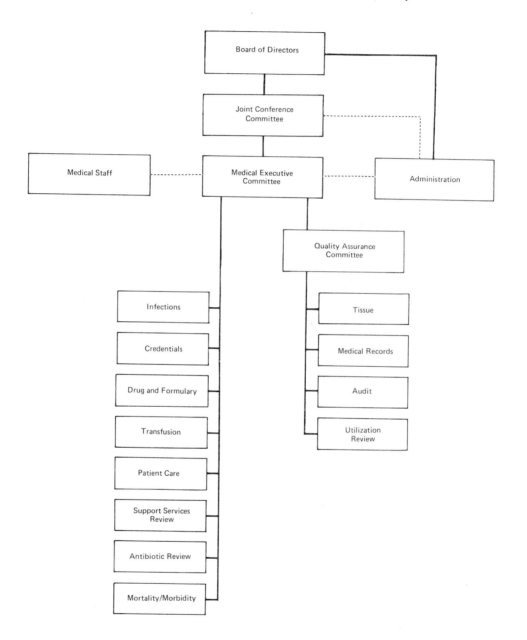

Completed Assessment Matrix, Hospital D

Assessment Questions	Credentialing	Clinical Department Review	Tissue/Surgical Case Review and Evaluation	Morbidity/Mortality	Pharmacy and Therapeutics	Blood Utilization Review and Evaluation	Antibiotic Usage Review and Evaluation	Nursing Care Review and Evaluation	Review and Evaluation of Support Services	Audit	Infection Control	Safety	Utilization Review	Risk Control	Continuing Education	Accreditation	Patient Representative Information
1. Is the function performed by an individual or committee?	C	C	C	C	C	C	C	I	C	C	C	C	Both	I	C	C	I
2. Who is routinely responsible for the function?	Chairman	Chairman	Chairman	Chairman	Chairman	Chairman	Chairman	Dept head	Chairman	Chairman	Chairman	Chairman	UR coord	VP	Dept heads	CEO	Dept heads
3. Is there a written description or procedure for the function?	Yes	Yes	~Yes	Yes	No	No	No	No	Yes	Yes	Yes	No	Yes	Limited	Yes	Yes	No
4. What data sources are used to perform this function?	Application	MRs	OR, TRs	TRs, death certificates	MRs, pharmacy logs	?	IC reports	Varies	?	MRs	Varies	Policies and procedures	MRs	Incident reports	?	Varies	Pt interviews
5. Are preestablished, clinically valid criteria used?	Yes	Yes	Yes	No	No	No	No	No	Yes	Yes	No	No	Yes	No	No	Yes	No
6. If a purpose of the function is to identify problems, are important problems identified?	Yes / No	Yes / Yes	Yes / No	Yes / No	Yes / No	Yes / ?	No / ?	No	No / ?	Yes / ?	Yes / ?	Yes / ?	Yes / ?	No / ?	No / ?	No / ?	? / ?
7. Does the responsible individual or committee recommend or implement action?	Both	R	Both	Both	Both	Both	Both	Both	Both	Both	Both	Both	Both	R	Both	Both	R
8. Is there monitoring to determine effectiveness of action?	No	Yes	No	No	Yes	No	No	No	No	No	No	No	No	No	No	No	?
9. To whom are the results of the function reported? With whom are they shared?	MEC, board / ?	Exec comm, board / ?	QAC / ?	EVP / ?	MEC / ?	Audit comm, admin / ?	IC / ?	EVP / ?	Dept heads / ?	QAC / ?	MEC / ?	Admin / ?	QAC, board / ?	VP / ?	MEC, dept heads / ?	Board / ?	Vp for pt serv / ?
10. Is the function evaluated routinely?	Yes	No	Yes	No	No	No	No	Yes	No	Yes	Yes	Yes	Yes	No	Yes	Yes	No

C=committee
CEO=chief executive officer
EVP=executive vice president
I=individual
IC=infection control

MEC=medical executive committee
MR=medical record
OR=operating room
Pt=patient
QAC=quality assurance committee

R=recommends
TR=tissue report
UR=utilization review
VP=vice president
?=do not know

Proposed Quality Assurance Plan for Hospital D

Hospital D will provide optimum quality care within available resources at a reasonable cost. To this end, Hospital D will develop a comprehensive integrated QA program and monitor all aspects of patient care within the institution. Every effort will be made to assure adequate sources of information to assist committees in the evaluation process. Monitoring patient care and taking action to correct deficiencies are vital to any QA program. No program can be complete, however, without effective follow-up that tracks the action taken and assures that the goals and objectives of the program have been reached.

Although peer review is a major factor in any QA program, the main intent in monitoring patient care activities is to assure that optimum quality of care is given to patients. Toward this end, the QA plan seeks to monitor all patient care activities and recommend change effectively (where appropriate).

Ancillary services should be provided only when appropriate. Optimum utilization of ancillary services will avoid unnecessary use of resources. Conversely, underutilization may not provide physicians with sufficient information to treat patients properly.

All professional staff clinical privileges will be reviewed annually. Input from all quality review activities will be used to assure that privileges are commensurate with clinicians' actual practice and abilities.

Surgical procedures will be reviewed to assure that proper documentation supports the need for surgery and that the diagnosis and surgical outcome is supported by appropriate clinical and ancillary tests.

Any QA program is incomplete without proper documentation. Every medical record should be sufficiently detailed to provide a running account of the patient's hospital stay. The process and outcome of patient care should be adequately reflected in each record.

Goals and Objectives

Mortality rates. Efforts will be made to reduce mortality rates to the lowest acceptable level. Of course death cannot be totally avoided, but the hospital's intent is to minimize mortality rates.

Length of stay. Patients should only remain in the hosptial for as long as they require acute medical care. To avoid unnecessary days of care or readmission due to early discharge, efforts will be made to have an optimal outcome.

Patient satisfaction. Impressions that patients have about the quality of care they receive often have little to do with the actual care provided. Patients with a positive attitude toward their care have an increased probability of positive outcomes. The hospital will therefore make an effort to address patients' nonmedical needs in hopes of improving patient satisfaction and impression of care.

Infections. Nosocomial infections delay patient improvement and increase utilization of medical resources. The hospital will make every effort to minimize nosocomial infections.

Patient treatment. Every effort will be made to assure that patients receive proper medications, treatments, and therapies.

Organization

The responsibility and authority for quality assurance ultimately lies with the board of directors, which delegates this responsibility to the joint conference committee. Composed of members of the board of directors, administration, and medical staff, the joint conference committee delegates ongoing monitoring of quality assurance to the medical staff which, through a series of committee activities, carries out the QA functions. Listed below are the committees involved in quality assurance, their responsibilities, and their representation. (See also the proposed organizational chart on page 167 and the flow of information chart on page 168.)

The joint conference committee has overall responsibility for quality assurance and is composed of members of the board of directors, administration, and medical staff.

The medical executive committee represents the medical staff in all areas involving patient care and, on behalf of the medical staff, is responsible for reviewing care. It is composed of members of the full-time medical staff and attending medical staff.

The quality assurance committee is responsible for coordinating all QA activities, maintaining a common data source, and developing reports for the medical staff to the joint conference committee.

The medical audit committee is responsible for process and outcome studies related to specific identified problems not in the province of other committees. It is composed of the director of quality assurance; representatives from the medical staff, medical records, nursing, and hospital administration; and of representatives from other hospital departments on an ad-hoc basis.

The utilization review committee is responsible for reviewing utilization of hospital resources through concurrent and retrospective studies. These studies include, but are not limited to, study of LOS, use of ancillary services, and use of treatments and therapies. The committee is composed of the director of quality assurance and representatives from the medical staff, admitting, social work, nursing, and administration.

The medical records committee is responsible for review of medical records to assure proper and complete documentation. It is composed of the director of quality assurance and representatives from the medical staff, medical record department, nursing, and hospital administration.

The tissue committee is responsible for reviewing all surgical activity and is composed of surgeons on the medical staff and representatives from hospital administration.

The staff privileges committee is responsible for credentials review and recommendations for staff privileges and takes into consideration all pertinent external data and internal data generated from QA committees. It is composed of representatives from the medical staff and hospital administration.

The infection committee is responsible for review of and action on all patient care activities that involve potential infection. It is composed of representatives from the medical staff, housekeeping, pharmacy, engineering and maintenance, dietary, laundry and linen distribution, nursing, and hospital administration.

The safety committee is responsible for reviewing all activities that relate to the safety of hospital personnel, patients, and property. It is composed of various hospital department heads and members of the medical staff as appropriate.

The patient care committee is responsible for reviewing all procedures, materials, and supplies used in patient care. It is composed of representatives from the medical staff, infection control, nursing, and hospital administration, and of hospital department heads as appropriate.

The transfusion practices committee is responsible for review of proper use of blood and blood derivatives for transfusion and for stocking the blood bank. The committee is concerned with education of house-staff and medical staff in the economical, proper, and safe use of blood and is composed of representatives from the medical staff, laboratory staff, nursing, and hospital administration.

The formulary and drug committee is responsible for reviewing and maintaining the hospital formulary, for collecting data for studying and tabulating drug reactions, for advising the medical staff on matters concerning the pharmacy and the dispensing of drugs, and for making recommendations on the proper storage and dispensing of investigational drugs when appropriate. It is composed of representatives from the medical staff, laboratory, pharmacy staff, nursing, and hospital administration.

Individual medical departments are routinely involved in QA activities that are in addition to hospital-wide committees with specific responsibilities for categorical components of patient care. Problems that relate specifically to a particular department will be reviewed and analyzed by department members and fed back to the QA committee. Questions on medical education that relate to quality of care will be reviewed by the individual departments, chiefs of service, or the education committee of the organized medical staff. When jurisdiction of assignments is questioned, decisions will be made by the QA committee and followed up by the specific committee involved.

Quality Assurance Committee

Program implementation will be the responsibility of the QA committee, which will conduct follow-up and assure that adequate and appropriate resources are used to uncover potential problems and that proper communication and authority lines are followed. The committee will assure that proper review components are used, such as resources, problem identification, establishing problem priorities, criteria development, performance measurement, deficiency analysis, action, and follow-up.

Information generated from each committee will be gathered and a centralized report on all QA activities will be developed. Identified problems and committee actions will be reported to the appropriate individuals and committees so they can carry out the responsibilities outlined in the plan. Every effort shall be made to keep all QA information and activities confidential, except where prohibited by law.

Members of hospital administration will staff various committees and provide appropriate resources to assist the committees to perform their duties. The QA department, through its director, shall provide the support and staff necessary to gather information and conduct studies.

Quality Assurance Department

Many QA activities involve overlapping and interrelated components. If several committees have interrelated responsibilities for the same problems, a centralized coordinating department should keep track of the entire process. The QA committee retains the overall responsibility for implementing the QA program, but the day-to-day activities of gathering data, assessing problems, recommending studies to the QA committee, and monitoring the entire process require a competent full-time staff.

Headed by the director of quality assurance, this department will have full-time or part-time staff (as required) responsible for gathering data; interpreting data; formulating recommendations for appropriate data review; conducting various studies, audits, and reviews; and providing staff support for the QA committee and all other committees involved in quality assurance. The department will be composed of individuals with data retrieval and review skills, statistics, knowledge of medicine and medical terminology, and other general skills as required.

The department will report to a member of hospital administration who will sit on each QA committee. The main purpose of the department is to assist all QA committees in carrying out their responsibilities.

Evaluation of the Quality Assurance Program

The plan shall be evaluated on an ongoing basis to assure that it meets the QA needs of the institution. At least annually, the plan shall be reviewed and revised if necessary by the QA committee, with input and assistance from other committees, medical departments, hospital departments, and the director of quality assurance. The medical staff and the joint conference committee will approve revisions and changes.

Proposed Organizational Chart, Hospital D

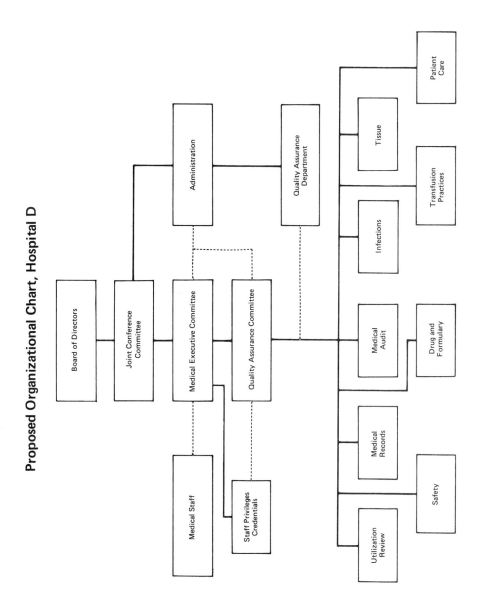

Illustration of Flow of Quality Assurance Information, Hospital D

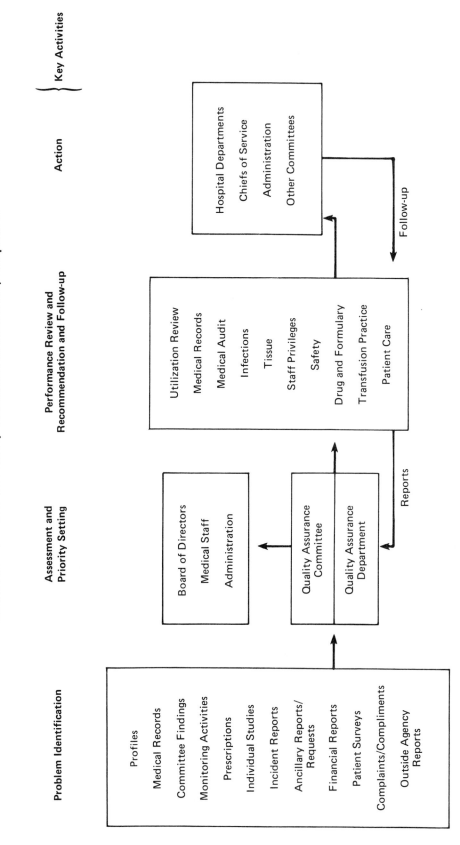

Hospital E: University Affiliated Hospital

A 998-bed hospital with university affiliation, Hospital E employs 500 house officers and approximately 200 active, full-time medical staff. Only limited clinical privileges are given to outside consulting physicians. Approximately 37,000 inpatients and 300,000 outpatients are seen at the hospital annually.

The governing body is composed of county commissioners and private citizens from business and civic sectors and was created in response to governance deficiencies cited by JCAH. The president of the governing body is CEO of the institution, is a member of the medical executive committee, and sits on the joint conference committee. The dean of the medical school is a member of the medical executive committee and also sits on the joint conference committee.

Three individuals report directly to the president of the governing body: the director of administrative services, the director of hospital operations, and the comptroller. Distinct hospital centers report to the director of patient services within operations.

Quality Assurance Activities in 1979

Hospital E has conducted organized QA activities for the past five years. The administrator for quality assurance is responsible for hospital-wide QA activities and has line responsibility for the infection control department, PSRO/UR activities, and the medical records department. A professional staff assistant reports to the administrator, coordinates accreditation and licensure activities, and ascertains that all documentation is current. Medical and multidisciplinary audit and UR requirements have been met for several years by a staff of ten, which includes nurses and medical record personnel. Three members of that staff coordinate 12 annual audits and required reaudits, and assist special subcommittees appointed by the chief(s) of service to set criteria. Topics are selected by the medical care evaluation committee, which approves all completed audits. Recommendations on corrective actions are discussed and passed on to the medical executive committee for action. Summaries of audits are presented to a committee of the governing board on a quarterly basis.

Meeting JCAH standards is considered extremely important, and accreditation is given high priority. The medical director of the QA program is salaried and oversees QA activities on a part-time basis.

Many QA activities are conducted simultaneously throughout the institution. Most noteworthy are those performed in nursing services and conducted by the nurse training and education department. The nurse educators participate with staff nurses at the unit level in a nursing process audit developed by Medicus. Results of these audits are shared only with the nursing service.

Other QA activities are conducted in many ancillary services but are not consistently reported to the patient care evaluation committee or to the QA department.

Analysis of the Assessment Matrix

Using the completed assessment matrix on the opposite page, Hospital E staff identified the following problems in their QA program:
- medical staff committees do not share results with nursing or ancillary service committees;
- authority for implementing action is lacking;
- some committees are not using preestablished, written criteria when appropriate;
- a definition of quality assurance is lacking in the institution;
- lines of accountability and communication need to be clarified;
- QA activities within departments and within the entire program are separate, distinct, and fragmented;
- varying degrees of importance are attributed to quality assurance by disciplines/services/departments within the institution;
- an insufficient understanding of activities that are appropriate and useful in a QA program exists; and
- results/findings of any activities are not shared.

Completed Assessment Matrix, Hospital E

Assessment Questions	Credentialing	Clinical Department Review	Tissue/Surgical Case Review and Evaluation	Morbidity/Mortality	Pharmacy and Therapeutics	Blood Utilization Review and Evaluation	Antibiotic Usage Review and Evaluation	Nursing Care Review and Evaluation	Review and Evaluation of Support Services	Audit	Infection Control	Safety	Utilization Review	Risk Control	Continuing Education	Accreditation	Patient Representative Information
1. Is the function performed by an individual or committee?	C	Both	C	Both	C	C	C	C	C	C	C	C	C	I	Various	?	I
2. Who is routinely responsible for the function?	Chairman	Dept head, comm	Chairman	Dept head	Chairman	Chairman	Chairman	Chairman	Chairman	Chairman	Chairman	Chairman	Chairman	I	Dept head	?	I
3. Is there a written description or procedure for the function?	Yes	Yes	Yes	Yes	Yes	Yes	Yes	Yes	Yes	Yes	Yes	Yes	Yes	Yes	Yes	?	Yes
4. What data sources are used to perform this function?	Application, references	Various	Tissue reports, MRs	M/M reports, MRs	Profiles, MRs	Transfusion reports	Pharmacy logs, MRs	MRs	MRs, logs	MRs	MRs, lab slips	IRs	MRs, admission documents	MRs, IRs	NA	?	MRs, interviews
5. Are preestablished, clinically valid criteria used?	Yes	Yes	Yes	NA	No	Yes	Yes	Yes	Yes	Yes	Yes	No	Yes	No	No	?	No
6. If a purpose of the function is to identify problems, are important problems identified?	No / ?	Yes / Yes	Yes / ?	Yes / ?	Yes / ?	Yes / ?	Yes / ?	Yes / ?	? / ?	Yes / ?	Yes / ?	Yes / ?	Yes / ?	Yes / ?	Yes / ?	? / ?	Yes / ?
7. Does the responsible individual or committee recommend or implement action?	R	Both	R	R	I	R	Both	R	R	R	Both	Both	R	Both	NA	?	R
8. Is there monitoring to determine effectiveness of action?	?	Yes	Yes	No	Yes	Yes	Yes	Yes	Yes	Yes	Yes	Yes	No	Yes	No	?	Yes
9. To whom are the results of the function reported? With whom are they shared?	MEC	?	MEC	QAC	MEC	MEC	IC, P&T	JCC, pt care	UR comm, pt care	JCC, pt care	MEC	JCC	JCC	EVP	JCC, pt care	?	Director pt serv
10. Is the function evaluated routinely?	?	Yes	?	?	?	?	?	?	?	?	?	?	?	?	?	?	?

C=committee
EVP=executive vice president
I=individual or implements
IR=incident report
JCC=joint conference committee
MEC=medical executive committee
M/M=morbidity/mortality
MR=medical record
PCC=patient care committee
Pt=patient
P&T=pharmacy and therapeutics
QAC=quality assurance committee
?=do not know

Proposed Quality Assurance Plan for Hospital E

Hospital E is mandated to provide patient care of high quality and to evaluate the quality of care and clinical performance provided. A QA program will be created to assure that this evaluation is performed.

The governing board has overall responsibility for the QA program and delegates authority to the medical executive committee, which delegates authority to the QA committee. Authority and delegation of authority for quality assurance are established in accordance with medical staff bylaws and rules and regulations.

Quality assurance refers to those activities or program components designed to evaluate patient care and identify, study, and correct deficiencies found in the patient care process. It shall consist of physician, nurse, and/or ancillary service review or systems interaction analysis; utilize objective criteria; provide recommendations; and allow for follow-up and/or reassessment.

Quality Assurance Committee

All hospital clinical services will be represented on the QA committee. Representatives from nursing service and QA administration will also serve. Suggested constituents include the medical director of quality assurance, an associate director of the hospital, the administrator of quality assurance, and committee chairpersons from the safety committee, the infection control committee, the pharmacy and therapeutics committee, the credentials committee, the ambulatory services committee, the medical records subcommittee, the tissue subcommittee, the cancer subcommittee, and the nursing clinical practice committee. Other professional personnel shall include the director of professional services and those department heads representing, but not limited to, respiratory therapy, radiology, anesthesia, the operating room, pathology, social services, and dietary services.

Purpose. The committee will oversee efforts to assure the highest possible quality of patient care through the analysis, review, and evaluation of clinical practices and support services throughout the hospital. It will determine the appropriate allocation of resources necessary to provide efficient and high quality patient care, and maximize utilization of staff and data sources to accomplish these goals.

Functions. The committee will consist of subcommittees responsible for the review of nursing practices; critical incidents; tissue, blood, and antibiotic utilization review; medical records; bed utilization; and problems identified throughout the hospital. Other medical staff or hospital-based activities may be considered in determining available data sources.

The committee will meet monthly at an appointed time. When necessary, special meetings may be called at the discretion of the chairperson.

The administrator of quality assurance will provide professional and clerical staff with expertise in quality assurance; adequate physical facilities and budgetary needs; and liaison to other hospital departments.

Other professional review. The departments of radiology, pathology, ambulatory services, infection control, social services, anesthesia, pharmacy, dietary services, and the operating room and other professional disciplines/services will be required to participate in QA activities through peer review, problem identification and resolution, and other methods as defined in the plan. Each will report at least quarterly to the QA committee and to the administrative representative who oversees departmental activity.

Committee reports and records. The minutes of all regular and special meetings of the QA committee will include the name of the committee or subcommittee; the date and duration of the meeting; the names of the committee members (present and absent) and guests; a description of activities presently in progress; and results, conclusions, status, and implementation of recommendations. Recommendations and reports are to be signed by the committee chairperson and forwarded to the executive committee and the governing body as deemed necessary. The committee will have the support of the administrative staff in assembling data, facilitating record review, and providing technical expertise when appropriate.

Quality Assurance Department

The QA department will use the following data sources to recommend areas for study to the QA committee: statistical reports from census data; reports from medical record discharges; incident reports; mortality and morbidity conferences; grand rounds conferences; utilization review findings; PSRO statistics; monitoring activities; patient care audits; financial data; patient surveys and patient representative reports; drug profile analyses; reviews of clinical services; hospital committee reports; data obtained from staff interviews and observation of hospital activities; and other sources that might prove beneficial to the QA program.

Evaluation of the Quality Assurance Program

The effectiveness of the QA program will be assessed semiannually and presented formally at the May and November meetings of the QA committee and to the joint conference committee of the governing body. Staff will prepare a report that compares annual goals and objectives to accomplishments. A sequential display of information will highlight items in progress and the extent of accomplishments. The summary of problems and corrective actions will be discussed and approved, when appropriate. The committee will vote to continue the program or to accept any alterations, additions, or deletions based upon documented activities. The summary of problems and corrective measures shall be approved by the executive committee, the CEO, and the governing body.

Proposed Table of Organization for Quality Assurance, Hospital E

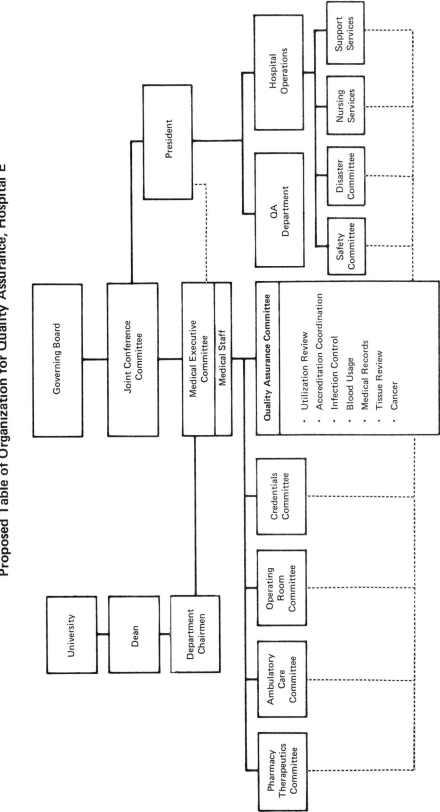

Appendix B.
Case Study Assessments

The case study assessments provided in this appendix are designed to assist the reader to further analyze the five case studies provided in Appendix A. The assessments are based on the Guidelines for Assessing a Quality Assurance Plan shown below. The case study assessments demonstrate further that the plans are published for illustrative purposes only and do not necessarily reflect compliance with the QA requirements of JCAH. Development of a QA plan is the responsibility of each hospital, and each plan should be specific to the needs of the individual hospital.

Guidelines for Assessing a Quality Assurance Plan

The following questions are designed to assist you in the development of a new, and/or in the assessment of an existing, QA plan.

Scope and Integration

1. *Are all disciplines that provide patient care represented in QA activities?*
2. *Who is responsible for the administration/coordination of the overall QA program?*

Problem Identification

3. *What activities and data sources are used to identify problems?*
4. *Who conducts each of these problem identification activities?*
5. *How frequently is each activity conducted and reported?*
6. *To whom is each activity reported and how is the information used?*

Priority Setting

7. *Who sets priorities for problem assessment and resolution?*
8. *Is there a mechanism for periodically updating priorities?*
9. *If priorities are not set centrally within the hospital, but are set on a departmental basis, is there a mechanism for central review and approval?*

Problem Assessment

10. *Who assesses identified problems?*
11. *Are predetermined, clinically valid criteria used to identify and assess problems?*
12. *To whom are results reported and how frequently are they reported?*

Problem Resolution

13. *Who is responsible for implementing action or resolution?*
14. *How frequently are the results of the action reported and to whom are they reported?*

Problem Monitoring/Follow-Up

15. *Who is responsible for monitoring problem resolution?*
16. *To whom are monitoring results reported?*

Evaluation

17. *How frequently is the program evaluated?*
18. *Who conducts the annual evaluation?*
19. *Through what mechanism is the program evaluated?*
20. *To whom are the results reported?*

Hospital A

Scope and Integration

1. *Are all disciplines that provide patient care represented in QA activities?*
   Yes, as outlined on the organizational chart and specified in the plan.
2. *Who is responsible for the administration/coordination of the overall QA program?*

The QA committee and the QA coordinator will administer and coordinate the program.

Problem Identification

3. *What activities and data sources are used to identify problems?*
   The plan does not specify data sources that will be used to identify problems.
4. *Who conducts each of these problem identification activities?*
   Activities are decentralized; responsibilities are assigned to appropriate committees and departments.
5. *How frequently is each activity conducted and reported?*
   The frequency with which each activity is conducted and reported is not specified.
6. *To whom is each activity reported and how is the information used?*
   Reports from each QA activity are sent to the QA committee for coordination and for action recommendation.

Priority Setting

7. *Who sets priorities for problem assessment and resolution?*
   The plan does not define who will set priorities.
8. *Is there a mechanism for periodically updating priorities?*
   The plan does not define whether a mechanism for setting priorities exists.
9. *If priorities are not set centrally within the hospital, but are set on a departmental basis, is there a mechanism for central review and approval?*
   The plan does not address centralization of the activity.

Problem Assessment

10. *Who assesses identified problems?*
    Problem assessment is conducted by each committee and each department.
11. *Are predetermined, clinically valid criteria used to identify and assess problems?*
    The plan does not specify if criteria will be used to identify and assess problems. This information may be contained in guidelines referenced in the plan.
12. *To whom are results reported and how frequently are they reported?*
    Results of problem assessment are sent to the QA committee, but frequency of reporting is not specified.

Problem Resolution

13. *Who is responsible for implementing action or resolution?*
    The chief of staff and the assistant executive director are responsible.
14. *How frequently are the results of the action reported and to whom are they reported?*
    Results of implemented actions are reported to the chief of staff and the assistant executive director, but frequency is not specified.

Problem Monitoring/Follow-Up

15. *Who is responsible for monitoring problem resolution?*
    The plan is not clear regarding who has responsibility for monitoring problem resolution. It could be the responsibility of the QA committee, the chief of staff and assistant executive director, or the departments and committees.
16. *To whom are monitoring results reported?*
    Follow-up reports are mentioned, but it is not clear who receives the reports, and frequency of reporting is not specified.

Evaluation

17. *How frequently is the program evaluated?*
    The program will be evaluated annually.
18. *Who conducts the annual evaluation?*
    The QA coordinator and the QA committee will conduct the evaluation.
19. *Through what mechanism is the program evaluated?*
    The effectiveness of the program will be measured by the problem identified, the actions taken, and the resolution of identified problems.
20. *To whom are the results reported?*
    Results of evaluation will be sent to the medical staff, administration, and the committees and departments. The organizational chart illustrates a reporting relation to the governing board (see page 139).

Hospital B

Scope and Integration

1. *Are all disciplines that provide patient care represented in QA activities?*
   Yes (see Proposed Quality Assurance Chart, page 147).
2. *Who is responsible for the administration/coordination of the overall QA program?*
   The QA coordinator is responsible.

Problem Identification

3. *What activities and data sources are used to identify problems?*
   The activities of the medical, nursing, and other professional staffs are delineated in the plan, but specific data sources are not specified.
4. *Who conducts each of these problem identification activities?*
   QA activities are decentralized, with each department having specific responsibilities.
5. *How frequently is each activity conducted and reported?*
   The frequency with which each activity is conducted has been identified on the organizational chart (see page 147). Specified time frames presumably apply to reporting as well.
6. *To whom is each activity reported and how is the information used?*
   Problems and identification information is reported to the QA coordinator, chief of staff, CEO, governing body, and appropriate clinical director. The QA coordinator uses the information to minimize duplication, and to coordinate resources and activities.

Priority Setting

7. *Who sets priorities for problem assessment and resolution?*
   The medical staff sets priorities (see pages 144 and 145).
8. *Is there a mechanism for periodically updating priorities?*
   The plan does not define a mechanism for updating priorities.
9. *If priorities are not set centrally within the hospital, but are set on a departmental basis, is there a mechanism for central review and approval?*
   Hospital B sets priorities through the medical staff.

Problem Assessment

10. *Who assesses identified problems?*
    Problem assessment is decentralized.
11. *Are predetermined, clinically valid criteria used to identify and assess problems?*
    Yes. Each discipline develops screening criteria to monitor problem identification/resolution and criteria to assess a specific problem.
12. *To whom are results reported and how frequently are they reported?*
    Results are documented in committee minutes and sent to the QA coordinator, medical staff, CEO, and governing body. Frequency is not specified.

Problem Resolution

13. *Who is responsible for implementing action or resolution?*
    Each discipline has responsibility for resolving problems; the chief of staff and the CEO provide support.

14. *How frequently are the results of the action reported and to whom are they reported?*
The results of action are reported to the QA coordinator, the medical staff, the CEO, and the governing body (see page 145). Frequency is not specified.

Problem Monitoring/Follow-Up

15. *Who is responsible for monitoring problem resolution?*
The medical staff is responsible for problem resolution (see page 146).
16. *To whom are monitoring results reported?*
Monitoring results are reported through the QA coordinator to the medical staff, the CEO, and the governing body.

Evaluation

17. *How frequently is the program evaluated?*
The program will be evaluated at least annually.
18. *Who conducts the annual evaluation?*
The governing body and the medical staff will conduct the annual evaluation.
19. *Through what mechanism is the program evaluated?*
The program will be evaluated annually by the governing body and the medical staff to ensure comprehensiveness, minimum duplication, and cost-effectiveness, and to ensure that important problems were identified and resolved.
20. *To whom are the results reported?*
The plan does not identify the recipient of evaluation results.

Hospital C

Scope and Integration

1. *Are all disciplines that provide patient care represented in QA activities?*
Although all disciplines are represented on the organizational chart, only medical staff activities are defined in the plan (see page 157).
2. *Who is responsible for the administration/coordination of the overall QA program?*
A multidisciplinary committee, the QA board, has responsibility for coordinating the program.

Problem Identification

3. *What activities and data sources are used to identify problems?*
   Criteria will be established to monitor each function.
4. *Who conducts each of these problem identification activities?*
   Various committees and departments are responsible for problem identification.
5. *How frequently is each activity conducted and reported?*
   The frequency with which each activity is conducted is not specified in the plan.
6. *To whom is each activity reported and how is the information used?*
   Results of activities are reported to the QA board and used to coordinate activities, establish priorities, and conduct monitoring.

Priority Setting

7. *Who sets priorities for problem assessment and resolution?*
   The QA board sets priorities.
8. *Is there a mechanism for periodically updating priorities?*
   The QA board would probably update priorities, but this responsibility is not specified in the plan.
9. *If priorities are not set centrally within the hospital, but are set on a departmental basis, is there a mechanism for central review and approval?*
   Priorities are set centrally.

Problem Assessment

10. *Who assesses identified problems?*
    Problems are assessed by the various departments and committees involved in QA activities.
11. *Are predetermined, clinically valid criteria used to identify and assess problems?*
    Criteria will be used to identify and assess problems.
12. *To whom are results reported and how frequently are they reported?*
    Results of problem assessment are reported to the QA board, but frequency of reporting is not specified.

Problem Resolution

13. *Who is responsible for implementing action or resolution?*
    The quality assurance board forwards recommended action to the appropriate authority for implementation.

14. *How frequently are the results of the action reported and to whom are they reported?*
The status of resolution of identified problems is reported to the QA board, but frequency of reporting is not specified.

Problem Monitoring/Follow-Up

15. *Who is responsible for monitoring problem resolution?*
The QA board is responsible (see page 154).
16. *To whom are monitoring results reported?*
Monitoring results are reported through the QA board to the medical executive committee and the board of directors.

Evaluation

17. *How frequently is the program evaluated?*
The program will be evaluated on an ongoing basis.
18. *Who conducts the annual evaluation?*
Each activity will evaluate its own QA effort.
19. *Through what mechanism is the program evaluated?*
The effectiveness of the overall program will be measured by achievement of established goals and objectives.
20. *To whom are the results reported?*
Evaluation results are reported, through the QA board, to the medical staff executive committee, the CEO, and the board of directors.

Hospital D

Scope and Integration

1. *Are all disciplines that provide patient care represented in QA activities?*
The plan is not comprehensive because it defines only the medical staff role in quality assurance.
2. *Who is responsible for the administration/coordination of the overall QA program?*
Coordination of the program is through the QA committee and the QA department. Committee composition is not specified in the plan.

Problem Identification

3. *What activities and data sources are used to identify problems?*
The activities conducted by the medical staff and the data sources

that will be used are identified in the Illustration of Flow of Quality Assurance Information (see page 168).

4. *Who conducts each of these problem identification activities?*
   Activities identified in the plan will be conducted by various committees and by the QA department.
5. *How frequently is each activity conducted and reported?*
   Frequency is not specified.
6. *To whom is each activity reported and how is information used?*
   Results are reported through the QA department to the QA committee. The QA department coordinates information.

Priority Setting

7. *Who sets priorities for problem assessment and resolution?*
   Responsibility for setting priorities is not stated clearly in the plan; it could be the QA committee, or the CEO/medical staff/board of directors (see pages 164 and 166).
8. *Is there a mechanism for periodically updating priorities?*
   This is not identified in the plan.
9. *If priorities are not set centrally within the hospital, but are set on a departmental basis, is there a mechanism for central review and approval?*
   Responsibility for setting priorities is not stated clearly.

Problem Assessment

10. *Who assesses identified problems?*
    Medical staff committees will assess problems related to the medical staff with assistance from the QA department. This has not been defined for nursing and support services.
11. *Are predetermined, clinically valid criteria used to identify and assess problems?*
    The QA committee will ensure that criteria are used by each activity.
12. *To whom are results reported and how frequently are they reported?*
    Results are reported to the QA committee through the QA department, but frequency of reporting is not specified.

Problem Resolution

13. *Who is responsible for implementing action or resolution?*
    Problem resolution is the responsibility of the appropriate authority and of the hospital departments, the chief of staff, the CEO, and various committees.

14. *How frequently are the results of the action reported and to whom are they reported?*
    Results are reported to the QA committee through the QA department, but frequency of reporting is not specified.

Problem Monitoring/Follow-Up

15. *Who is responsible for monitoring problem resolution?*
    The various committees will monitor problem resolution.
16. *To whom are monitoring results reported?*
    Results are reported to the QA committee through the QA department, but frequency of reporting is not specified.

Evaluation

17. *How frequently is the program evaluated?*
    The program will be evaluated on an ongoing and annual basis.
18. *Who conducts the annual evaluation?*
    The QA committee will conduct the evaluation with input from other committees, medical and hospital departments, and the director of the QA department.
19. *Through what mechanism is the program evaluated?*
    The plan does not specify how the program will be evaluated.
20. *To whom are the results reported?*
    Results of the evaluation will be reported to the medical staff and the joint conference committee.

Hospital E

Scope and Integration

1. *Are all disciplines that provide patient care represented in QA activities?*
   Yes. The plan includes medical, nursing, and support services (see Proposed Table of Organization, page 175).
2. *Who is responsible for the administration/coordination of the overall QA program?*
   The QA committee, with assistance from the QA department, is responsible for coordination of the QA program.

Problem Identification

3. *What activities and data sources are used to identify problems?*
   A variety of data sources will be used.

4. *Who conducts each of the problem identification activities?*
   Problem identification has been decentralized; responsibility is shared by the QA committee, the QA department, clinical departments, and by other committees such as the safety committee, etc.

5. *How frequently is each activity conducted and reported?*
   The QA committee will conduct monthly meetings; QA department activities will be continuous; and the other activities will be reported at least quarterly.

6. *To whom is each activity reported and how is the information used?*
   Results are reported to the medical staff and administration through the QA committee and other committees. Such results will be used to coordinate information, including data sources, and to determine staff and resource allocation (see Proposed Table of Organization, page 175).

Priority Setting

7. *Who sets priorities for problem assessment and resolution?*
   This may be a function of the QA committee, but a plan for priority setting is not specifically defined.

8. *Is there a mechanism for periodically updating priorities?*
   See response to Question 7.

9. *If priorities are not set centrally within the hospital, but are set on a departmental level, is there a mechanism for central review and approval?*
   See response to Question 7.

Problem Assessment

10. *Who assesses identified problems?*
    Each committee and department is responsible.

11. *Are predetermined, clinically valid criteria used to identify and assess problems?*
    Criteria will be used, but the use of and responsibility for developing criteria is not defined. (A statement in the plan regarding the use of criteria is not required.)

12. *To whom are results reported and how frequently are they reported?*
    Results are reported quarterly to the QA committee and the appropriate administrative representative.

Problem Resolution

13. *Who is responsible for implementing action or resolution?*
    The QA committee is responsible for implementing and monitoring action for its primary activities. The activity has been decentralized,

and each clinical department is responsible for implementing and monitoring action.

14. *How frequently are the results of action reported and to whom are they reported?*

    Action results are reported quarterly to the QA committee.

Problem Monitoring/Follow-Up

15. *Who is responsible for monitoring problem resolution?*

    Monitoring activities are not delineated nor are requirements for frequency of reporting.

16. *To whom are monitoring results reported?*

    See response to Question 15.

Evaluation

17. *How frequently is the program evaluated?*

    The plan specifies semiannual evaluation.

18. *Who conducts the annual evaluation?*

    The staff of the QA department will assist the QA committee.

19. *Through what mechanism is the program evaluated?*

    The program's success will be measured by its ability to meet annually established goals and objectives. Whether goals and objectives will be hospital-wide or department-specific is not delineated, nor is responsibility for developing goals and objectives.

20. *To whom are the results reported?*

    Results are reported to the medical staff, the executive committee, the CEO, and the joint conference committee of the governing body.

Appendix C.
Selected Assessment Methods

The specific quality assessment techniques considered in this appendix include the Comprehensive Quality Assurance System (CQAS), Concurrent Quality Assurance (CQA), Criteria Mapping, Generic Screening, Health Accounting, Performance Evaluation Procedure (PEP), Problem Status Index–Outcome (PSI), Quality Assurance Monitor (QAM), Staging, Sentinel Health Events, Tracers, and the CMA/CHA Patient Care Audit. These methods, which are described only briefly, were selected as a representative sample of a vast number of available assessment methods. Their selection is not intended to imply endorsement by the Joint Commission on Accreditation of Hospitals, which has emphasized flexibility in its quality assurance standard. The standard is designed to encourage application of a wide range of assessment strategies, selected and implemented on the basis of individual need and/or the type and extent of problems under consideration.

Developed by individuals or organizations as mechanisms for assessing the quality of care, these methods differ from one another in the extent of refinement, ease of implementation, applicability, and usefulness of results. Because none of these methods necessarily is problem-focused, they need to be modified by hospitals and expanded to become applicable as problem-focused methods. When selecting an assessment method, consider the characteristics of the problem to be assessed, the strengths of various assessment methods, and the specific components of the methods which might be useful during assessment of a particular problem(s).

Comprehensive Quality Assurance Systems (CQAS)*

Developed for the Northern California Kaiser-Permanente Medical Centers, CQAS is based on the use of single criteria to identify highly suspicious problems. Using microsampling techniques and implicit standards, two practitioners review a small number of records to identify problems in patient care. Results of this review are presented to a quality assurance committee which, in turn, selects the most important suspected problems for further assessment and then sets explicit standards of care based on these problems. For example, "The record will show that all children will have proper immunization therapy by the age of five years or documentation of the reasons why they have not been immunized," or "All chest x-rays revealing abnormalities not specified as old will have been followed up or have a note referring to x-ray or x-ray report."

These standards become the criteria for a document-based review, which is used to evaluate current compliance. Records that do not comply with the standards are reviewed by a physician who, using implicit standards for quality care, determines whether problems in care exist. Corrective actions are implemented when actual problems are determined. The problem is reassessed to determine whether it has been resolved or, at least, reduced to an acceptable level.

This method encourages involvement of a large number of physicians or other health care professionals and provides for both problem identification and assessment. According to this method, problem identification is a careful, two-part process. However CQAS relies heavily, if not exclusively, on process criteria and document-based information. Further, because of its reliance on several levels of physician or practitioner review, the method can be costly and time-consuming.

Concurrent Quality Assurance (CQA)†

Private Initiative in PSRO (PIPSRO) tested a method of concurrent quality assurance that is now used to examine the technical quality of care for specific diagnoses while patients are still under treatment. For each selected diagnosis, a panel of experts predetermines process criteria for the following three categories: diagnostic criteria, which specify the objective data required to substantiate the diagnosis; documentation criteria, which stipulate that information be entered in the record on co-

---

*Rubin L, Kellogg MA: The comprehensive quality assurance system. In Giebink GA, White NH, Short ES (eds): *Ambulatory Medical Care Quality Assurance.* La Jolla, CA: La Jolla Health Sciences Publications, 1977, pp 141-167.

†Sanazaro PJ, Worth RM: Concurrent quality assurance in hospital care: Report of a study by private initiative in PSRO. *N Eng J Med* 298:1171-1177, 1978.

morbidity, on predisposing or etiological factors, on stage or severity of the condition, and on the presence or absence of complications that modify treatment or prognosis; and treatment criteria, which indicate the optimal process of treatment for the diagnosis. Immediate outcomes that can reasonably be expected as a result of treatment are also defined and posted prominently in the records of participating patients.

Adherence to all criteria is assessed on a *concurrent* basis so that corrective action, when indicated, can be implemented immediately.

Although CQA stresses resolution of problems as they occur (presumably to the benefit of both current and future patients), the assessment is disease-oriented, and problems in care that are more generic are not assessed easily.

Criteria Mapping*

Criteria mapping is a document-based review that tracks practitioner logic in the clinical decision-making process. A diagram (decision tree) of the numerous sequential decisions that should be made in a specific clinical situation is developed (see pages 199 and 201 for examples of such diagrams). Potential alternative decisions are provided at each decision step (node on the tree). Criteria (alternate clinical decisions) that assist one to reach these predetermined decisions appear on the decision tree as nodal points and continue to branch out and track each step in the decision process. The branching format enables application of only those criteria and decisions that relate to a specific patient, and helps determine which branch of the criteria map is applicable and what subsequent actions or decisions should be taken. Compliance with criteria can be assessed at each decision step.

Criteria mapping attempts to account for the specificity and complexity of each patient rather than aggregating patients by disease category or diagnosis. Criteria maps applied to clinical records provide assessment of a group of clinicians or patients, and the method can be used successfully by most disciplines.

Generic Screening†

In 1977, the California Medical Insurance Feasibility Study assessed the number and severity of potentially compensable events, without regard

---

*Kaplan SH, Greenfield S: Criteria mapping: Using logic in evaluation of processes of care. *QRB* 4:3-9, Jan 1978.

†Mills DH: Report of the California Medical Insurance Feasibility Study. California Medical Association/California Hospital Association (unpublished), 1977.

to legal fault, that could be attributed to medical management. In this study, 20 generic criteria were developed that could be applied to all diagnoses and clinical problems. These criteria were used for risk management purposes, that is, identification of potentially compensable events that also are indicators of potential problems in patient care. (For an illustration of these criteria, see pages 68-69.)

Considering such items as readmission, mortality, hospital-incurred trauma, and adverse drug reaction, generic criteria can be used to identify possible problem areas. Once problems are identified, evaluation and assessment of their causes, as well as corrective actions and appropriate reassessment, should be initiated.

*Medical Management Analysis,** a risk management system, was developed based on generic screening criteria. A professional liability warning system, it provides a flexible, centralized framework for comprehensive, concurrent review of all patient records and immediate follow-up of hospital-incurred adverse events and patterns of substandard care.

Generic screenings are used for concurrent document-based review and are relatively efficient, inexpensive, and flexible (criteria other than the original 20 can be used). They can be used by all disciplines and the problems they identify are likely to have significant adverse impacts. On the other hand, generic screening is not a high yield assessment method as events screened by these criteria do not occur frequently and the criteria are not designed to elicit much information about the probable sources (causes) of a problem.

Health Accounting†

Developed in collaboration with 23 hospitals and clinics throughout the United States, Health Accounting is a five-stage approach to quality assurance, which involves several steps. Included in these steps are the following:

- formulation of priorities from an extensive list of nominated study topics, using structured group judgment** and a team of generalists appointed from within the hospital;
- estimation by the team, using structured group judgment tech-

---

*Craddick JW: The Medical Management Analysis System: A professional liability warning mechanism. *QRB* 5:2-8, April 1979.

†Williamson JW: *Assessing and Improving Health Outcomes—The Health Accounting Approach to Quality Assurance.* Cambridge, MA: Ballinger, 1978.

**Delbecq A, Van de Ven A, Gustagson D: *Group Techniques for Program Planning: A Guide to Nominal Group and Delphi Process.* Glenview, IL: Scott, Foresman and Co, 1975.

niques, of the amount of impact likely to be achieved by study of selected high priority topics;

- verification of the existence and extent of impact of the problems (by a specially trained evaluation assistant) and determination of the seriousness of its impact in terms of health or economic outcomes;
- identification of correctable determinants of the verified problem, using more definitive evaluation studies;
- final planning and implementation of a formal effort to resolve identified problems; and
- use of the original assessment to remeasure and determine whether problems have been resolved or reduced to an acceptable level.

Health Accounting is a flexible, outcome-oriented assessment method that uses all available data from all sources and seeks additional data if necessary. It is intended to be a quality assurance system rather than a limited assessment technique. Health Accounting is, however, a sophisticated quality assurance system that requires experienced, trained staff who have problem-solving skills. Outside technical consultation often is required to establish the system.

Performance Evaluation Procedure for Auditing and Improving Patient Care (PEP)*

The PEP system is an outcome-oriented, retrospective method of review that uses preestablished criteria to evaluate patient care by reviewing patient records selected on the basis of a common diagnosis or procedure. The system may be adapted to verify the existence of a problem and determine its extent and probable causes. The method focuses on hospital care, is defined by such parameters as validation of diagnosis, justification for admission, justification for surgery or special procedures, discharge outcomes, complications and critical management for complications, length of stay, and, sometimes, charges. Although outcome-oriented, the method allows inclusion of critical process criteria and is useful in evaluating patterns of data. Once criteria are established for an audit, data retrieval and display can be implemented by nonphysicians. (For an example of an area-wide audit based on the PEP method, see pages 202-208.)

---

*Joint Commission on Accreditation of Hospitals: *The PEP Primer.* Chicago: Joint Commission on Accreditation of Hospitals, 1974.

Problem Status Index-Outcome (PSI)*

Although it can be used to assess the outcomes of inpatient care, PSI is used primarily to assess the outcomes of ambulatory care from the patient's point of view. Questionnaires are sent to patients at a predetermined time after contact with a health care provider. The timing of the questionnaire is determined by the clinical problem and its expected patient outcomes. The questionnaire is designed to elicit patients' perceptions about the frequency and severity of symptoms and limitations imposed on their activity. These perceptions about health status are compared to expected outcomes of acceptable care by correlating patients' reported outcomes with process information in the medical records.

The development of PSI questionnaires can be complex and expensive, and the response rate can be low. However, PSI is one of the few methods that focuses on patient's perceived experiences with therapeutic intervention and on outcomes of care beyond those that occurred in the hospital.

Quality Assurance Monitor (QAM)†

Developed by the Commission on Professional and Hospital Activities (CPHA), QAM is a continuous monitoring technique that attempts to provide reasonable surveillance of patient care. The system is also a priority-determination technique used to signal areas that may require more detailed study. QAM-3 monitors various parameters of care for three groupings within a hospital: hospital-wide groups, department-wide groups, and diagnosis-specific and surgery-specific groups. The hospital receives a priority-for-investigation listing which compares the hospital's performance with standards set by professional organizations and with the performance of all other Professional Activity Study facilities in the hospital's region. The priority-for-investigation listing also indicates possible problem areas that may require in-depth study.

The quality assurance monitor offers rapid assessment of many areas on which a hospital might focus quality assurance activities and offers comparisons to other similar hospitals. However, QAM is a screening system only, and any priority-for-investigation requires detailed assessment to verify the existence, extent, and probable source of a problem.

---

*Mushlin AI: An experimental mechanism for quality assurance in a prepaid group practice. In *Proceedings of the Group Health Institute*. Washington: Group Health Association of America, 1974. And Mushlin AI et al: Quality assurance in primary care: A strategy based on outcome assessment. *J Com Health* 3:292-305, 1978.
†Lowe JA: PASport. *QRB* 3:20-23, Aug 1977.

Staging*

An outcome-based assessment method developed to assess ambulatory care and modified for inpatient use, Staging is used to determine the patient's status upon entering the hospital; measures change in that status over time; and separates health problems into three levels of severity—conditions with no complications or minimal severity, local complications or moderate severity, and systemic complications or maximal severity. Quality of care is assessed by the extent of change in stage associated with medical intervention and, to some extent, accessibility is measured by the patient's stage at admission to the hospital (or entrance to the health care system). The distribution of stages for the patient population being studied can be compared to standards for comparable populations.

Staging is one of the few assessment methods that takes case mix severity into consideration early in the problem identification process. However, staging is useful only for screening disease-oriented problems in care and may not be particularly sensitive to subtle quality of care problems even in the disease categories under study.

Sentinel Health Events†

Sentinel Health Events are negative health events including unnecessary disease, unnecessary disability, and untimely death. A negative index of health is developed by measuring the incidence of these three general types of events. The purpose of this kind of assessment is to focus on preventable or treatable conditions to ascertain if they are being prevented or treated effectively or, conversely, if there are problems in the care provided to patients.

This type of assessment focuses on outcomes and is most useful as a screening device for problem identification. However, it is very difficult to set standards for acceptable levels of unnecessary disease and disability, and measurement of the incidence of Sentinel Health Events assumes diagnostic accuracy that may be questionable. The data produced from this assessment relate to incidence rates, not the probable cause of the problem.

---

*Gonnella JS, Cattani JA, Louis DZ et al: Use of outcome measures in ambulatory care evaluation. In Giebink GA, White NH, Short ES (eds): *Ambulatory Medical Care Quality Assurance.* La Jolla, CA: La Jolla Health Science Foundation, 1977, pp 91-125.

†Rutstein D, Berenberg W, Chalmers TC: Measuring the quality of medical care. *N Eng J Med* 294:582-588, 1976.

Tracers*

Tracers originally were developed to evaluate care provided by a neighborhood health center. The author states that one can make judgments regarding the functioning of an entire health care system by assuming that the care provided for certain tracer health problems is representative of care in general. Each of these tracers could shed light on how certain elements of the system work—not in isolation, but in relation to other elements. Tracers attempt to focus evaluation activity on both process and outcome aspects of care that will provide the most useful information regarding the quality of care. Once appropriate tracer conditions are identified, criteria for each condition are formulated. These criteria are set at minimally acceptable levels, focus on pragmatic rather than technologically sophisticated care, are subject to periodic revision, and apply to general populations rather than specific patients. Criteria are established for appropriate screening techniques, essential elements of the patient's history and physical examination, necessary lab tests, and evidence of appropriate diagnosis and management.

CMA/CHA Educational Patient Care Audit†

A form of traditional medical audit, the CMA/CHA Patient Care Audit has two unique features not found in other methods of medical audit. That is, the CMA/CHA audit requires that physicians be substantially involved in their own evaluation by ratifying the criteria by which they will be evaluated and by setting "thresholds for action." Thresholds indicate the minimum percentage of records which must meet preestablished criteria before care can be considered acceptable. These thresholds, unless set too high, encourage efficiency because they define problems for which correction is needed and because they define the extent of problem resolution (below threshold) that can realistically be achieved.

---

*Kessner DM, Kalk CE, Singer J: Assessing health quality: The case for tracers. *N Eng J Med* 288:189-194, 1973.

†CMA/CHA: *Educational Patient Care Audit Manual.* San Francisco: California Medical Association/California Hospital Association, 1975.

Examples of Assessment Methods

Example 1. *Study of Microscopic Hematuria*

The study of microscopic hematuria, shown on pages 198 and 199, illustrates the use of criteria mapping (or algorithms) as assessment methods. Criteria mapping helps track practitioner logic in the clinical decision-making process. The physician collects preliminary patient data, identifies positive findings, and makes decisions about or takes action on the next step of care based on these findings. Used as assessment methods, algorithms or criteria maps help assess whether or not practitioners provided care that was appropriate to a specific patient, taking into account variations of a specific diagnosis. That is, the branching format of an algorithm or criteria map addresses the processes of symptom evaluation and longitudinal care while simultaneously accounting for patient specificity and case complexity.

Example 1. *Study of Microscopic Hematuria*

Nondelegated Focused Study

Topic	Hematuria
Sample	Three-month retrospective sample, from April 1, 1979, to January 1, 1979. Up to 25 charts; include all federal patients.
Perceived Problem	Red blood cells in the urine are often overlooked in routine urinalysis; further investigation is not always conducted.
Objective	To determine if the presence of red blood cells in the urine, on routine urinalysis, is investigated.
Methodology	Medical care evaluation staff will collect information on a retrospective basis through use of an algorithm. Every medical record in which a routine urinalysis is filed will be included in the screening process. Each urinalysis will be checked to determine if the presence of red blood cells was recorded.
	Data will be aggregated and analyzed by the medical review committee. A decision will be made regarding further commitment of resources to the study of this topic.
Results	19 charts were found to have abnormal routine urinalyses. Based on justifiable exclusions noted on the algorithm, 4 charts were excluded from the study. 7 of the 15 charts remaining in the study did not demonstrate completion of the algorithm for microscopic hematuria. These charts will be submitted to the committee for discussion.

Example 1. (continued)   *Study of Microscopic Hematuria*

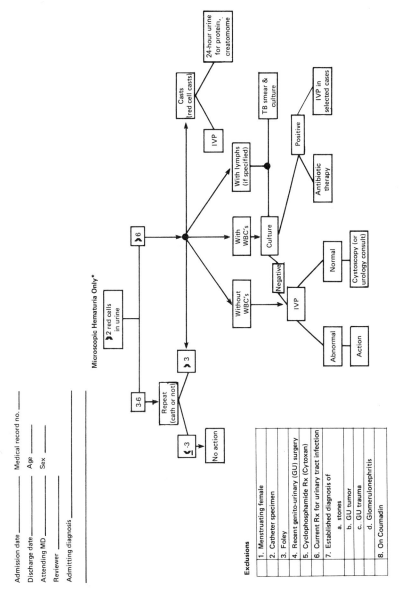

Admission date _____   Medical record no. _____

Discharge date _____   Age _____

Attending MD _____   Sex _____

Reviewer _____

Admitting diagnosis _____

Microscopic Hematuria Only*

>2 red cells in urine

Repeat (cath or not)

No action

Casts (red cell casts)

24-hour urine for protein, creatomome

IVP

With lymphs (if specified)

TB smear & culture

Positive

IVP in selected cases

Antibiotic therapy

With WBC's

Culture

Without WBC's

Negative

IVP

Normal

Cystoscopy (or urology consult)

Abnormal

Action

Exclusions

1. Menstruating female
2. Catheter specimen
3. Foley
4. Recent genito-urinary (GU) surgery
5. Cyclophosphamide Rx (Cytoxan)
6. Current Rx for urinary tract infection
7. Established diagnosis of
a. stones
b. GU tumor
c. GU trauma
d. Glomerulonephritis
8. On Coumadin

*Gross hematuria requires immediate cystoscopy

Example 2. *Observation Study**

A nursing study of patients with chest tubes (see page 201) adapted the concept of criteria mapping to an observation study. Nurses developed a protocol that used branching logic to determine whether chest tubes are patent and draining and whether patients have signs or symptoms of complications resulting from chest tube insertion.

This particular algorithm is probably more useful as an educational tool in the proper procedure for chest tube care. Although time-consuming to develop, a protocol based on algorithms is easy to implement, serves a wide variety of assessment and teaching functions, and is relatively inexpensive.

---

*Harper RW, Rhodes MA: Development and application of flow charting techniques in nursing practice. JONA 7:5, 17, May/June 1977. Reprinted with permission.

Example 2. *Observation Study*

Section of a Flow Chart Entitled
"Care of the Patient with Chest Tubes"

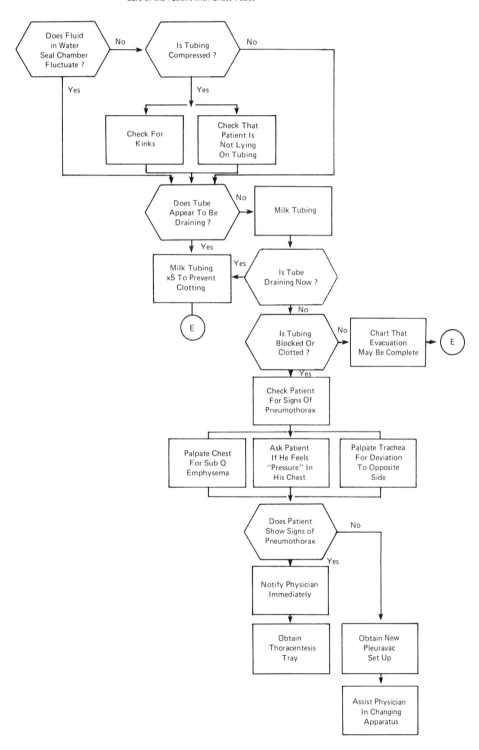

Example 3. *Area-Wide Medical Evaluation Study**

An area-wide or multihospital medical care evaluation study can be an excellent tool for in-depth exploration of a problem that is perceived as common within a geographic area or among several hospitals and that could have a significant health and economic impact. An area-wide or multihospital audit is a lengthy procedure which requires extensive overall management of communication and implementation of the audit among hospitals. Clinically valid criteria must be established that are acceptable to and that work for each hospital that is involved. Extensive amounts of data must be collected and analyzed, and results must be communicated in a manner that preserves confidentiality as well as fosters the maximum potential for learning.

Area-wide audits can, therefore, be cumbersome and time-consuming. On the other hand, an area-wide study might actually decrease the amount of time and resources expended by any one facility. Such studies also permit comparisons by hospital. These comparisons can be enhanced if regional and national norms are also displayed so that hospitals can compare themselves with hospitals throughout a region.

The study of blood utilization shown on the following pages is interesting in that it compares rates of justified and unjustified variations (see page 207) and displays the numbers of decisions with which additional physician reviewers agreed and disagreed (see page 208).

---

*Washington State Professional Standards Review Organization Area-Wide Medical Care Evaluation Study, Topic Area—Generic Audit on Transfusions, Specific Topic—Transfusions, Jan 12, 1978. Printed with permission.

Example 3. *Area-Wide Medical Evaluation Study**

Title Audit Study Specifications on the Topic of Transfusions

Study Objectives

To assure that correct utilization of blood and blood products occurred and that the desired effects of the transfusion were obtained.

Index codes	
H-ICDA	**ICDA-8**
94.6	R9.1
94.7	74.1

Includes: Extraoperative

Excludes: Intraoperative

Alternative Methods for Records Identification

1. Examine the list of units of blood signed out from hospital blood bank.
2. Track prospectively, until appropriate sample size is obtained, all records containing evidence that a blood transfusion was given.

Recommended Guidelines for Selecting Sample Size

Admissions per year	Under 500	500-2000	2000+
Minimum no. of records	(50)	(75)	(100)

In hospitals with more than 50 beds, 20% of the cases should be surgical and 80% nonsurgical.

---

*Washington State Professional Review Organization Area-Wide Medical Care Evaluation Study, Topic Area--Generic Audit on Transfusions, Specific Topic--Transfusions.

Example 3. (continued)   *Area-Wide Medical Evaluation Study*

Criteria Development Worksheet

Audit Topic: Transfusion (excluding intraoperative)

Elements	Standard 100%	Standard 0%	Exceptions	Definitions and Instructions for Data Retrieval
Justification for Transfusion (one or more)				
1. Hypovolemia due to acute blood loss	X		1A. Patients admitted for renal dialysis	1. **Hypovolemia.** Acute blood loss, described in record as extraoperatively from a particular site and 24 hours prior to transfusion; or blood loss described at time of surgery with one of the following:
			1B. Patients with Hb of <10g or Hct <30% who require major surgery under general anesthesia	a. CVP <30mm/H_2O.
OR				b. Systolic blood pressure 90mm/Hb or less and/or pulse rate of 120/min or greater.
				c. Hct <30% or 25% postpartum.
Chronic anemia				**Chronic anemia.** Hg <6.5gm/100ml or Hct 20% or less.
OR				**Anemia syndrome.** Pulse >100/min and/or respiration >30/min, and/or dizziness, fainting, weakness and Hct 25% or less **or** Hb 8.5 gm or less.
Anemia syndrome				
OR				Committee to review all transfused pernicious anemias, iron deficiency anemias, and malabsorption syndromes.
Exchange transfusion				**Exchange transfusion.** In newborns only; committee to see all others.
Key Elements of Management				
2. Vital signs taken before, during, and after transfusion*	X		2. None	2. See vital signs or graphic record and nurses notes.

*Nursing criterion

Example 3. (continued) *Area-Wide Medical Evaluation Study*

Criteria Development Worksheet

Elements	Standard 100%	Standard 0%	Exceptions	Definitions and Instructions for Data Retrieval
Discharge Status				
3. Hct > 30%	X		3. None	3. See lab reports.
4. Systolic blood pressure >100mm/Hg (in any position)	X		4. Patient less than 12 years of age	4. See graphic sheet or nurses' notes.
5. Free of hypotensive symptoms	X		5. Physician aware of symptoms and makes notation in progress notes	5. Blood pressure falls and patient gets dizzy or faints when sitting or standing up. See MD's progress notes or discharge summary and nurses' notes.
6. Mortality		X	6. None	
Other				
7. Single unit tranfusion during hospitalization.		X	7. Patient less than 15 years of age	7. Unit = 450-500 ml.
8. More than 7 units of blood given		X	8. None	8. See transfusion record, nurses' notes, and MD's progress notes.
9. Whole blood given		X	9A. Packed cells not available	9A. See transfusion requisition form.
			9B. More than 1,000 ml of acute blood loss	9B. See admission notes, MD's progress notes.
			9C. Signs and symptoms of hypovolemia as defined in no. 1	
10. Readmission to this hospital within eight months of any patient with hepatitis, syphilis, malaria, or hemosiderosis			10. None	10. Committee to review all charts.

Example 3. (continued)   *Area-Wide Medical Evaluation Study*

Criteria Development Worksheet

Elements	Standard 100%	Standard 0%	Exceptions	Definitions and Instructions for Data Retrieval
Complications				
11. Circulatory overload		X	11. None	11. Patient develops cough, shortness of breath, or cyanosis during transfusion. See MD's progress notes or nurses' notes.
12. Febrile reaction		X	12. None	12. Rise temperature by 1° C (1.8° F) during or within 30 minutes of transfusion.
13. Bacterial contamination of donor blood		X	13. None	13. See discharge diagnosis for bacteremia/septicemia and look for positive blood culture. *Committee to review all charts.*
14. Transfusion reaction (red cell incompatibility)		X	14. None	14. See MD's progress notes and nurses' notes. *Committee to review all charts.*
15. Allergic reaction		X	15. None	15. Development of hives or rash during transfusion. See MD's progress notes or nurses' notes. *Committee to review all charts.*
16. Anaphylaxis		X	16. None	16. Blood pressure drops 30mm/Hg or more during transfusion, wheezing, laryngospasm, hives, and/or facial edema. See MD's progress notes and nurses' notes.

Note: Committee to review complications 11-16 for appropriateness of critical management.

Example 3. (continued) *Area-Wide Medical Evaluation Study*

Area-Wide Transfusion Audit: 1978
Variation Display by Criterion*

Criterion	Justified Variations	Unjustified Variations
1. Justification	479	284
2. Vital signs †	150	1080
3. Hct ›30%	299	100
4. Systolic BP ›100mg/HG	154	133
5. Free of hypotensive symptoms	52	60
6. Mortality	136	8
7. Single unit transfusions	89	83
8. ›7 units of blood	86	6
9. Whole blood	241	245
10. Readmit within 8 months with hepatitis, syphilis, malaria, or hemosiderosis	3	2
Complications		
11. Circulatory overload	10	7
12. Febrile reaction	141	33
13. Bacterial contamination	5	2
14. Transfusion reaction	20	15
15. Allergic reaction	44	14
16. Anaphylaxis	9	2
17. Other complications	6	7

* Statewide totals: 2396 records
† Nursing criterion

Example 3. (continued)　*Area-Wide Medical Evaluation Study*

Area-Wide Transfusion Audit: Eastern District (Reviewer's Analysis)

Hospital Number

	1	2	3	4	5	6	7	8	9	10	11	12	13	14	15	16	17	18
Number of records	50	50	100	55	100	50	40	63	100	47	47	50	45	75	100	43	75	45
Justified variations	62	24	99	38	164	39	5	64	91	24	58	55	29	64	96	7	73	23
Unjustified variations	81	35	82	21	124	51	21	44	148	70	50	26	32	137	120	6	218	89
Total	143	59	181	59	288	90	26	108	239	94	108	81	61	201	216	13	291	112
Reviewer's Analysis																		
Agreed with variation analysis rationale	143	58	177	49	276	34	26	77	**	85	108	75	61	197	195	**	288	107
Disagreed with variation analysis rationale	0	1	4	9	11	4	0	11	**	8	0	6	0	4	21	**	3	5
Number of variations without documented rationale	0	0	0	1	1	1	0	20	**	1	0	0	0	0	0	**	0	0
Action appropriate	X	X	X	X	X	X	?	?	**	X	X	X	X	X	X	**	X	X
Plan for follow-up	X	X	X	X	X	X	?	?	**	?	X	X	X	X	X	**	X	X

Key:　X = yes
?. = questionable
** = insufficient information
　　to make a decision

Appendix D. Selected References on Quality Assurance

As the field of quality assurance has advanced and interest in the development and modification of quality assurance systems has increased, the number of useful, interesting publications has also increased. The references which are provided on the following pages are only a few of the excellent articles and publications which are now available on quality assurance and related topics.

Adeylotte MK: *Nurse Staffing Methodology: A Review and Critique of Selected Literature.* Iowa City: University of Iowa College of Nursing, Jan 1973.

Adler GS, Dobson A: The strategy of evaluating nationwide MCE impact. *QRB* 5:8-11, Oct 1979.

Avery AD, Lelah T, Solomon NE et al: *Quality of Medical Care Assessment Using Outcome Measures: Eight Disease-Specific Applications.* Santa Monica, Calif: Rand, R-2021/2HEW, 1976.

Barr DM, Gaus CR: A population based approach to quality assessment in Health Maintenance Organizations. *Med Care* 11:523-528, 1973.

Brook RH: *Quality of Care Assessment. A Comparison of Five Methods of Peer Review.* Washington, DC: National Center for Health Services Research and Development, Department of Health, Education and Welfare (DHEW), DHEW pub no. HRA-74-3100, Jul 1973.

Brook RH, Appel FA, Avery C et al: Effectiveness of inpatient follow-up care. *N Eng J Med* 285:1509-1514, 1971.

Brook RH, Berg MH, Schechter PA: Effectiveness of nonemergency care via an emergency room—A study of 116 patients with gastrointestinal symptoms. *Ann Intern Med* 78:333-339, 1973.

Brook RH, Stevenson RL: Effectiveness of patient care in an emergency room. *N Eng J Med* 283:904-907, 1970.

Cochrane AL: *Effectiveness and Efficiency.* London: The Nuffield Provincial Hospitals Trust, 1972.

Codman EA: *A Study in Hospital Efficiency: The First Five Years.* Boston: Thomas Todd, 1916.

Davis JB, Bader BS: The systems approach to patient safety. *QRB* 5:17-21, Feb 1979.

Dershewitz RA, Gross RA, Williamson JW: Validating audit criteria: An analytic approach illustrated by peptic ulcer disease. *QRB* 5:18-25, Oct 1979.

Diamond H, Luft LL: A selected bibliography of literature on quality assurance for community mental health centers. *QRB* 6:27-31, Apr 1980.

Dietz JW, Phillips JL: The quality assurance committee in the hospital structure. *QRB* 6:8-12, Jan 1980.

Donovan RJ Jr, Bader BS: The systems approach to patient safety: Role of the medical staff. *QRB* 5:16-20, Apr 1979.

Fessel WJ, VanBrunt EE: Quality of care and medical record. *N Eng J Med* 286:134-138, 1972.

Gonnella JS, Goran MJ: Quality of patient care—A measurement of change: The staging concept. *Med Care* 13, 1975.

Gonnella JS, Goran MJ, Williamson JW et al: Evaluation of patient care. *JAMA* 214:2040-2043, 1970.

Gonnella JS, Louis DZ, McCord JJ et al: Toward an effective system of ambulatory health care evaluation. *QRB* 3:7-9, Oct 1977.

Greene R: *Assuring Quality in Medical Care: The State of the Art.* Cambridge, Mass: Ballinger, 1976.

Haussman RD, Hegyvary ST: *Monitoring Quality of Nursing Care, Part 3: Professional Review for Nursing: An Empirical Investigation.* Washington, DC: GPO pub no. 017-022-00569-7, Aug 1977.

Horn BJ: *Criterion Measures of Nursing Care Quality.* Ann Arbor: University of Michigan, Department of Hospital Administration, NTIS pub no. PB-287-449-3, Aug 1978.

Horn SD, Roveti GC, Kreitzer SL: Length of stay variations: A focused review. *QRB* 6:6-10, Feb 1980.

Howe MJ, Coulton MR, Almon GM et al: Developing scaled outcome criteria for a target population. *QRB* 6:17-23, Mar 1980.

Howe MJ, Coulton MR, Almon GM et al: Use of outcome criteria for a target population. *QRB* 6:15-21, Apr 1980.

Institute of Medicine: Advancing the quality of health care; key issues and fundamental principles. Policy statement by a committee of the Institute of Medicine, National Academy of Sciences, Washington, DC, 1974.

Kaplan SH, Greenfield S: Criteria mapping: Using logic in evaluation of processes of care. *QRB* 4:3-7, Jan 1978.

Kessner DM, Kaik CE, Singer J: Assessing health quality — The case for tracers. *N Eng J Med* 288:189-194, 1973.

Kisch AI, Kovner JW, Harris LJ et al: A new proxy measure for health status. *Health Serv Res* 4:223-230, 1969.

Kisch AI, Reeder LG: Client evaluation of physician performance. *J Health Hum Beh* 10:51-58, 1969.

Lang NM: *Quality Assurance in Nursing: A Selected Bibliography.* Nurse Planning Series, DHEW pub no. HRA 80-30, Mar 1980.

Lembcke PA: Evolution of the medical audit. *JAMA* 199:111-118, 1967.

Lerner M, Riedel CD: The teamster study and the quality of medical care. *Inquiry* 1:69-80, 1964.

Logsdon DN: A selected bibliography of literature on ambulatory health care. *QRB* 5:22-27, Aug 1979.

Lyons TF, Payne B: The relationship of physicians' medical recording performance to their medical care performance. *Med Care* 12:463, 1974.

Mech AB: Evaluating the process of nursing care in long term care facilities. *QRB* 6:24-30, Mar 1980.

McNeil BJ, Varady PD, Burrows BA et al: Measures of clinical efficacy: Cost effectiveness calculations in the diagnosis and treatment of hypertensive renovascular disease. *N Eng J Med* 293(5):216-221, 1975.

Morehead MA: The medical audit as an operational tool. *Am J Public Health* 57:1643-1656, 1967.

Pauker SG, Kassirer JP: Therapeutic decision-making: A cost/benefit analysis. *N Eng J Med* 293:229-234, 1975.

Payne BC, Lyons TF, Dwarshins L et al: *Quality of Medical Care: Evaluation and Improvement.* Health Services Monograph Series T40. Chicago: Hospital Research and Education Trust, 1976.

Quality Review Bulletin (QRB): *Infection Control and Drug and Antibiotic Review.* Chicago: Joint Commission on Accreditation of Hospitals, 1979.

QRB: *Integration Issues in Quality Assurance.* Chicago: JCAH, 1980.

QRB: *Multidisciplinary Audit.* Chicago: JCAH, 1980.

QRB: *Nursing Audit.* Chicago: JCAH, 1978.

QRB: *Toward a Comprehensive Quality Assurance Program.* Chicago: JCAH, 1979.

Richardson FM: Peer review of medical care. *Med Care* 10:29-39, 1972.

Rosser RM, Watts VC: The measurement of hospital output. *Int J Epidemiol* 1(4):361-368, 1972.

Sanazaro PJ, Williamson JW: End results of patient care: A provisional classification based on reports by internists. *Med Care* 6:123-130, 1968.

Sanazaro PJ, Worth RM: Concurrent quality assurance in hospital care. *N Eng J Med* 298:1171, 1978.

Sapin SO, Borok GM, Tabatabai C: A region-wide quality of care monitoring and problem delineation plan. *QRB* 6:13-19, Feb 1980.

Schumacher DN, Stack K: MCEs refocused: Use of hospital resources by patients with congestive heart failure. *QRB* 4:15-18, Oct 1978.

Shapiro S: End result measurements of quality of medical care. *Milbank Mem Fund Quart* 45(2):127-150, 1967.

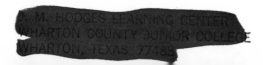

Starfield B: Measurement of outcome: A proposed scheme. *Milbank Mem Fund Quart* 52(1):39-50, 1974.

Stearns G, Fox LA: A three-phase plan for integrating quality assurance activities. *QRB* 6:13-16, Jan 1980.

Williamson JW: *Assessing and Improving Health Care Outcomes: The Health Accounting Approach to Quality Assurance.* Cambridge, Mass: Ballinger, 1978.

Williamson JW: Evaluating quality of patient care: A strategy relating outcomes and process assessment. *JAMA* 218:564-569, 1971.

Williamson JW: Formulating priorities for quality assurance activity— Description of a method and its application. *JAMA* 239:631-637, 1978.

Williamson JW, Alexander M, Miller GE: Priorities in patient-care research and continuing medical education. *JAMA* 204:303-308, 1968.

Williamson JW, Aronovitch S, Simonson L et al: Health accounting: An outcome based system of quality assurance: Illustrative application to hypertension. *Bull NY Acad Med* 51:727-738, 1975.

Williamson JW, Braswell HR, Horn SD et al: Priority setting in quality assurance: Reliability of staff judgment in medical institutions. *Med Care* 16:931-940, 1978.